On the Dark Side of Chronic Depression

This book brings together cutting-edge expertise from psychoanalysis, psychiatry, neuroscience and social science to shed light on the dark side of chronic depression.

Considering different forms of depression on a continuum, the book develops new diagnostical considerations on depression. It includes detailed case studies from clinical psychoanalytical practice, conceptual considerations and historical analyses to current empirical and neurobiological studies on depression. The book is unique in bridging a gap between Anglo-Saxon/German psychoanalysis and French traditions in relation to clinical treatment techniques and conceptualizations of depression and trauma. Chapters present new research on the social, biographical, genetic and neurobiological determinants of severe depressive disorder and explore how these can be differentiated and expanded in the face of new cultural realities as well of new findings, particularly in modern neurosciences.

The book explores new understanding and discussion of treatment options for depression and will be essential reading for researchers and students in the field of depression and mental health research. It will also enrich the conceptual and clinical knowledge of psychoanalysts and psychotherapy researchers and students.

Marianne Leuzinger-Bohleber is Professor Emeritus for psychoanalysis at the University of Kassel, past director in charge of the Sigmund-Freud-Institut in Frankfurt and now researcher at the Universitymedicine in Mainz, Germany.

Gilles Ambresin is Research Lead in the research program on chronic depression at the University Institute of Psychotherapy, Lausanne University Hospital, Switzerland.

Tamara Fischmann is Professor of clinical psychology and psychoanalysis at the International Psychoanalytic University (IPU) Berlin, Germany and researcher at the Sigmund-Freud-Institut (SFI) Frankfurt a.M.

Mark Solms is Chair of Neuropsychology at the University of Cape Town and Groote Schuur Hospital, South Africa.

Advances in Mental Health Research

Books in this series:

"This is a long-awaited book integrating psychoanalytic insights into chronic severe depression with progress that has been made in psychoanalytic and sociocultural research. It is an excellent and unique contribution which all clinicians will benefit from."

Peter Fonagy, Head of the Division of Psychology and Language Sciences at UCL; Chief Executive of the Anna Freud National Centre for Children and Families, London; Consultant to the Child and Family Programme at the Menninger Department of Psychiatry and Behavioural Sciences at Baylor College of Medicine; and holds visiting professorships at Yale and Harvard Medical Schools

"As the prevalence of depression grows, the need for better treatments is heightened. This volume provides an in-depth exploration of the psychodynamic and socio-cultural mechanisms of depression including new research on the role of early childhood trauma. I recommend this book to anyone who wishes to expand their understanding of depression beyond conventional approaches."

Richard D. Lane, MD, PhD, Professor of Psychiatry, Psychology and Neuroscience, The University of Arizona, USA

"Reading this book is an inspiring experience. A fresh approach is presented to the nature of chronic depression using modern interdisciplinary language. The book entails a promise of important new understanding of why the suffering of people with long-term depression has been so difficult to change. Highly recommendable."

Johannes Lehtonen, Professor of Psychiatry Emeritus, University of Eastern Finland; Adjunct Professor of Clinical Neurophysiology, University of Turku, Finland; Member of The Finnish Psychoanalytical Society

"A book for readers who sense the value of an in-depth integrated understanding of depression: how it is essential if an injured individual is to grow emotionally; and as well for all of us as creatures, each with our natures, histories, nationalities and cultures in the approaching global crisis of our species."

Dr David Taylor, Training & Supervising Analyst of the Institute of Psychoanalysis, London; Clinical Director of the Tavistock Adult Depression Study (TADS); Visiting Professor at UCL; and a trustee of the Melanie Klein Trust

"This book admirably shows why depression needs a psychoanalytic approach that goes beyond the symptoms and addresses the suffering human beings, their bodies and minds, their history and traumas, and their family and social life."

Ricardo Bernardi, Professor Emeritus at the School Medicine, Uruguay; "Honorary Member" ("Miembro de Honor") and Training Analyst of the Uruguayan Psycho-analytical Association (APU) and of the Uruguayan Society of Psychiatry; Full Member of the National Academy of Medicine, Uruguay; IPA Extraordinarily Meritorious Service to Psychoanalysis Award (2021); Mary S. Sigourney Award for Major Contribution to Psychoanalysis (1999); International Journal of Psychoanalysis (IJP) Best Paper Award (2003)

"This volume that originated in the work of the 2020 Joseph Sandler Conference in Lausanne offers readers at all levels of psychoanalytic experience a comprehensive, state-of-the-art exploration of an integrative model of depression seen from varying perspectives. These include empirical, metapsychological, social-scientific, research-based and clinical considerations. In doing so, it addresses core clinical issues of narcissism, trauma, intra-psychic and relational conflict and examines and exemplifies the important role of empirical research in psychoanalysis. The result is a much-valued resource for the understanding of the origins, presentations and treatment of depression in its many manifestations, that range from classical melancholia to essential depression and from neurosis to psychosis."

Howard B. Levine, Md, Editor-in-Chief, the Routledge
Wr Bion Studies Series

On the Dark Side of Chronic Depression

Psychoanalytic, Social-cultural and Research Approaches

Edited by
Marianne Leuzinger-Bohleber, Gilles Ambresin, Tamara Fischmann and Mark Solms

R Routledge
Taylor & Francis Group

LONDON AND NEW YORK

First published 2023
by Routledge
4 Park Square, Milton Park, Abingdon, Oxon OX14 4RN

and by Routledge
605 Third Avenue, New York, NY 10017

Routledge is an imprint of the Taylor & Francis Group, an informa business

British Library Cataloguing in Publication Data
A catalogue record has been requested for this book

ISBN: 978-1-032-24567-6 (hbk)
ISBN: 978-1-032-24568-3 (pbk)
ISBN: 978-1-003-27929-7 (ebk)

DOI: 10.4324/9781003279297

Typeset in Times New Roman
by Taylor & Francis Books

Contents

Figures

Contributors

Christine Anzieu-Premmereur is Professor in Psychiatry in the Department of Psychiatry of Columbia University College of Physicians and Surgeons and Director of the Parent–Infant Psychotherapy Training Program, Columbia University Center for Psychoanalytic Training and Research, New York, USA. She practices as a child psychoanalyst and is chair of the IPA COCAP, member of the APsaA, and the Société Psychanalytique de Paris. She publishes in scientific journals and has authored several book chapters.

Gilles Ambresin is Research Lead in the research program on chronic depression at the University Institute of Psychotherapy, Department of Psychiatry, Lausanne University Hospital, Switzerland. Associate member at the Swiss Psychoanalytic Society (SSPsa), psychiatrist and psychotherapist, practicing in private practice. Past member of the Board of the Centre de Psychanalyse de Lausanne, Chair of local organizing committee of the XXIst Sandler conference in Lausanne, Member of the organizing committee of the Congrès des psychanalystes de langue française (Lausanne, 2023). He publishes in peer-reviewed journals and authored book chapters focusing mainly on severe or chronic depression and psychotherapy. (ORCID: 0000-0001-8983-8501)

Valérie Bouville is past President of the German Psychoanalytic Association (2019–21). She is a medical doctor, psychiatrist and psychologist, training and supervising psychoanalyst and works in her own practice in Bonn, Germany. She is particularly interested in the relationship between language and the psyche and how different cultures impact our psychological development and identity and how psychological mechanisms are passed on from generation to generation.. She is an expert in bridging the French and German/Anglosaxon traditions in psychoanalysis und has made many translations. Her newest publications are: "The uncanny double" (2019) and "Zwischen Schuld und Trauma" (2020). (ORCID: 0000-0003-2713-5100)

Anne Brun, Lyon Director of the Research Centre for Psychopathology and Clinical Psychology, CRPPC, EA 653, at the Lumière Lyon 2 University. Professor 1st class, University of Lyon 2. Professor of Psychopathology and Clinical Psychology at the University of Lyon 2. Membre adhérent de la SPP. Doctorate in psychoanalytical studies at the University of Paris VII. Prof. Anne Brun has written more than 60 peer-reviewed articles, more than 80 book chapters and five scientific books, and edited nine scientific books. (ORCID: 0000-0003-4858-7050)

Nicolas de Coulon is Training Analyst and past President of the Swiss Psychoanalytical Society, former Board Member of the International Psychoanalytic Association (IPA) and past Member of the IPA Executive Committee. Past Medical Director of the Nant Foundation, psychiatric sector and hospital (Vaud East, Vevey-Montreux region). In addition to his clinical work as psychoanalyst, psychoanalytic psychotherapist and psychiatrist in private practice and his teaching and supervising functions, he is involved in the development of qualitative research methods in psychotherapy and psychoanalysis, in collaboration with Professor Jean-Nicolas Despland and Dr Bernard Reith. He has also published scientific and clinical articles, principally in psychoanalytic journals and reviews. (ORCID: 0000-0002-8199-2771)

Jean-Nicolas Despland is Psychiatrist and Psychotherapist, full member of the Swiss branch of the European Federation for Psychanalytic Psychotherapy (EFPP), host member of the Lausanne Psychoanalytic Centre of the Swiss Psychoanalytical Society, full professor at the Faculty of Biology and Medicine of the University of Lausanne and Director of the University Institute of Psychotherapy (IUP) of the Department of Psychiatry (CHUV, Lausanne). In addition to his clinical and training activity, he devotes himself to the study of the efficacy and processes in psychotherapy. This research is based on instruments allowing defense mechanisms, conflictual relational themes, the therapist's interventions, as well as the therapeutic alliance to be to assessed in a qualitative and quantitative way. Since 1998, he has enjoyed continuous support from the SNSF and others and has published more than 200 scientific and clinical articles, as well as several books. (ORCID: 0000-0002-5877-6616)

Tamara Fischmann is Professor of Clinical Psychology and Psychoanalysis at the International Psychoanalytic University (IPU) Berlin, Germany, practicing psychoanalyst DPV/IPA and staff member and scientific researcher at the Sigmund-Freud-Institut Frankfurt, Germany. Her publications mainly focus on interdisciplinary research in bioethics, dream research, attachment, as well as imaging technique studies in neurosciences. She is currently engaged in a project investigating the biological function of dreaming and in another project looking at the psychoanalytic and biological underpinnings of multiple complex traumatization in early childhood. (ORCID: 0000-0003-3990-8174)

Siri Erika Gullestad is Professor Emeritus of Clinical Psychology, University of Oslo, Norway and a training and supervising psychoanalyst. Gullestad is former dean of the Department of Psychology, University of Oslo, and former president of the Norwegian Psychoanalytic Society. For many years, she was the leader of Clinic for Psychodynamic Therapy, providing training in psychoanalytic psychotherapy for psychology students. She is an experienced teacher and supervisor. Gullestad is the author of numerous articles and books within the psychoanalytic field. Her latest book, co-authored with Bjørn Killingmo, is *The Theory and Practice of Psychoanalytic Therapy: Listening for the Subtext* (Routledge, 2020).

Silke Kratel Cañellas is Practicing Psychoanalyst, Member of the Swiss Psychoanalytic Society (SSPsa), Practicing Psychoanalysis and Psychotherapy for children, adolescents and adults, Children and Adolescent Psychiatrist, supervising consultant for the Office Medico Pédagogique in Geneva, Member of the Scientific Committee, Master in Psychoanalytic Psychotherapy.

Marianne Leuzinger-Bohleber is past Director in Charge of the Sigmund-Freud-Institut in Frankfurt a.M., Germany (2001–16), Professor Emeritus for Psychoanalysis at the University of Kassel, Senior Professor at the IDeA Excellency Center in Frankfurt a.M. and the University medicine in Mainz. She is training analyst of the German Psychoanalytical Association (DPV) and former member of the Swiss Psychoanalytical Society and the International Psychoanalytical Association. She is Chair of the Committee for Research and Universities of the (DPV), was 2001–09 Chair of the Research Subcommittees for Conceptual Research of the International Psychoanalytic Association (IPA); since 2010 she has been Vice Chair for Europe of the Research Board der IPA, and 2018–19 chair of the IPA Subcommittee for Migration and Refugees. (ORCID: 0000-0002-2421-2564)

Bernard Reith is Training Analyst and President of the Swiss Psychoanalytical Society for 2019–2022, past Chair of the Working Party on Initiating Psychoanalysis (WPIP) of the European Psychoanalytic Federation and presently Chair of the Working Parties Committee of the International Psychoanalytic Association, and Regional Editor for Europe of the *International Journal of Psychoanalysis*. In addition to his clinical work as psychoanalyst, psychoanalytic psychotherapist and psychiatrist in private practice and his teaching and supervising functions, he is involved in the development of qualitative research methods in psychoanalysis. He has co-edited *Initiating Psychoanalysis: Perspectives* (2012) and is co-author of *Beginning Analysis: Processes in Initiating Psychoanalysis* (2018). (ORCID: 0000-0002-4768-0889)

Jean-Claude Rolland works in private practice as psychoanalyst in Lyon, France. He is a referee to the *International Journal of Psychoanalysis* and past and founding editor of the *Libres cahiers pour la psychanalyse*. He is a full member of Association Psychanalytique de France, past Vice-President of the Board of the Association Psychanalytique de France, past President of the Board of the Association Psychanalytique de France, past member of the IPA working group on Borderline States, and past member of the IPA Board of representatives. He has authored several books and contributed to numerous book chapters. He also publishes in psycho-analytic journals.

Dominique Scarfone is Honorary Professor, Department of Psychology, Université de Montréal, Canada, MD (Psychiatry) and former training/supervising psychoanalyst. Recently retired member of the Canadian Psychoanalytic Society and Institute and of the International Psychoanalytic Association, he recently ceased his private practice in psychoanalysis and psychotherapy in Montreal. He has authored and edited books as well as book chapters on psychoanalysis. He has published more than 70 articles in peer-reviewed journals and is frequently invited as guest speaker in international psychoanalytic conferences. (ORCID: 0000-0002-5709-5077)

Daniel Schechter is currently Senior Consultant in Child and Adolescent Psychiatry and Medical Director of Perinatal and Early Childhood Research and Ambulatory Care at the Lausanne University Medical Center Child and Adolescent Psychiatry Service, Switzerland. He serves concurrently as Associate Professor of Psychiatry on the Faculty of Biology and Medicine at the University of Lausanne, and Adjunct Associate Professor of Child and Adolescent Psychiatry at the New York University School of Medicine. He is a faculty affiliate of the Columbia University Center for Psychoanalytic Training and Research in New York and the International Psychoanalytic University in Berlin. His original research has focused on the psychobiological impact of maternal history of interpersonal violence exposure on the caregiving environment during early childhood development, on parent–child psychopathology, intergenerational transmission of trauma, and related intervention. (ORCID: 0000-0003-1663-6305)

Jean-François Simoneau, Master in Psychology, is full member of the Swiss Psychoanalytical Society, full member of the European Psychoanalytical Psychotherapy Association, Chair of the organizing comity of the Congrès des Psychanalystes de Langue Française, CPLF 2022. Beside his clinical work as psychoanalyst, psychoanalytic psychotherapist for children, teenagers and adults in private practice in Lausanne, he is involved in teaching and supervising psychoanalysis and psychotherapy. He is a contributor to the book *Play and Primary Forms of Symbolization* (in press) (Dunod, 2020).

Mark Solms holds the Chair of Neuropsychology at the University of Cape Town and Groote Schuur Hospital, South Africa (Departments of Psychology and Neurology) and is a past president of the South African Psychoanalytical Association. He is also currently director of the American Psychoanalytic Association's science department. Solms is best known for his discovery of the forebrain mechanisms of dreaming, and for his integration of psychoanalytic theories and methods with those of modern neuroscience.

Gérard Winterhalter is psychiatrist and psychotherapist in private practice, certified member of the European Federation for Psychoanalytic Psychotherapy (past president of the Swiss section). In addition to his clinical activity and training in psychoanalytic psychotherapy, he has a long experience in practice and training in crisis intervention. He made a presentation and wrote a book chapter on the dynamics of prescription drugs in 2009.

Preface

The contributions in this volume are based on papers delivered at the Joseph Sandler Research Conference which took place in October 2020 at the University of Lausanne (Lausanne University Hospital). When we chose the topic of this international research conference we had no idea how much the title *On the Dark Side* would capture a core feeling of many of us during these months of the pandemic crisis. In a completely unexpected sharpness, many of the latent societal problems – the "dark sides" – have been washed to the surface. The Bulgarian philosopher Ivan Krastev expressed this as follows: "The crisis only brings out more clearly what was already there anyway. It is not the epidemics that change society, but they make us see the truth about our society .... We see what we could not see before" (Interview in *Spiegel*, 2.6.2020, p. 122, translation MLB).

The pandemic makes us all look into the abyss of the human psyche. This burdens all of us, psychoanalysts and analysands, politicians and citizens, members of all social and educational strata worldwide. The completely unexpected, elusive, uncontrollable danger to life, to which we have been exposed powerlessly – without medication or vaccine – confronted us with a situation of total dependence and powerlessness. From a psychoanalytical point of view, images of intubated people lying helplessly on their belly in intensive care units, for example, reactivate memories of ubiquitous early experiences in the first months of life. As is well known, an infant can only survive if it is sufficiently well cared for and looked after physically and psychologically. The infant is in an existential situation of total dependence. The embodied memories of these basic human experiences remain unconsciously in our memory and are reactivated, especially by the confrontation with death, throughout our lives.

It thus seemed inevitable that COVID 19 would also cast its shadow on the conference. We offered one panel on Saturday afternoon, where we reflected directly on the effects of the pandemic on clinical psychoanalytic work and, for example, discussed the question whether and in what way psychoanalysis as a science of the unconscious might contribute to the public and inter-disciplinary debates on dark sides of the pandemic. As the Italian Psycho-analytical Society has impressively shown, psychoanalysts can also be helpful offering crises interventions for traumatized people from the medical care sector, affected persons and relatives. Four hundred Italian colleagues were involved in these offers, especially in areas in Northern Italy most severely affected by the virus (see www.spiweb.it/cultura/ipa-society-community-initia tives-contributo-della-presidente-sul-covid/, see also the special issue of the *Journal of Applied Psychoanalytic Studies* 2020, on this topic). The specific psychoanalytic knowledge on acute and extreme trauma, but also on the (primitive) defense mechanisms triggered by them, such as denial, splitting, grandiose negation, projection and projective identification, as well as on the enactments of ubiquitous unconscious fantasies, may belong to genuine psychoanalytic contributions to the ongoing public discourses on the pandemic as well as the associated, perhaps even more threatening topic of climate change (Freud, 1931).

COVID 19 also shaped the format of the Sandler Conference 2020. It was the first Sandler Conference in a (hybrid) format with a mixture of virtual and in-person conference under strict hygiene rules. It was a tightrope walk for all of the participants not to deny the current danger due to COVID 19 on the one hand, but on the other hand not to be distracted too much by the pandemic and – in spite of all the dark sides during these months of the pandemic in society – to try to use the opportunity of the conference to gain a deeper clinical, conceptual and empirical understanding of the *subjective experiences of patients with chronic depression in a combination of psychoanalytic, neurobiological and socio-cultural perspectives.*

Multiperspective approaches to complex, relevant societal topics always have belonged to the central aims of the Sandler Conference. The Joseph Sandler Research Conference is the only exclusive research conference of the International Psychoanalytic Association (IPA). It was founded in 1990 by Joseph Sandler, Robert Wallerstein, Otto Kernberg, Robert Emde, Peter Fonagy and others to bring psychoanalysis out of the ivory tower and to address hot social issues from a psychoanalytic research perspective, by clinical, conceptual and empirical research. Another aim was to discuss empirical psychoanalytical research with clinicians, for research had existed in psychoanalysis from the very beginning, but often leads a shadowy existence or even triggers great ambivalence in the psychoanalytical community. The Sandler conferences thus aim at promoting and intensifying the dialogue between psychoanalytical researchers and clinicians.

A new specificity of the Sandler conference in Lausanne, taking place for the first time in a French-speaking region, was that we aimed to build a bridge between Anglo-Saxon/German psychoanalysis and French traditions, a bridge which, both in the European Psychoanalytic Federation (EPF) and in the IPA, posed particular challenges in terms of clinical treatment techniques, conceptualizations of depression and trauma and different attitudes towards empirical research. In this volume we are documenting some of the outcomes of this unique and interesting exchange.

We are grateful to many colleagues who helped us to organize the Sandler Conference under the difficult pandemic situation as well as to the local

professional groups which supported the organization from the very beginning. Our deep thanks to the Swiss Society of Psychoanalysis (President 2020,
Bernard Reith) and to the European Federation of Psychoanalytic Psychotherapy Suisse Romande (President 2020, Richard Simon). Without the
support of the Institute of Psychotherapy (Department of Psychiatry, Lausanne
University Hospital, Director Jean-Nicolas Despland) the holding of the conference would not have been possible. The International Psychoanalytic Association cannot support the Joseph Sandler Conferences financially but by
appreciating the activities of the International Research Board (IRB) (Chair in
2020, Mark Solms) normally combining the Research Training Program (RTP)
(Chairs in 2020, John Clarkin, Robert N. Emde) with the Joseph Sandler
Research Conference (responsible in 2020, Marianne Leuzinger-Bohleber, Vice-
Chair of the IRB in 2020). After intensive discussion we decided to cancel the
RTP in 2020 due to the pandemic. We are grateful for the shared responsibility
with the chairs of the RTP and the local organizing Committee (Chair, Gilles
Ambresin). Finally, we would like to extend our gratitude to the invaluable help
of members of staff (Audrey Desbonnet, Eileen Rabel and Delphine Genoud)
who made the conference run smoothly.

Marianne Leuzinger-Bohleber, Gilles Ambresin, Tamara Fischmann
and Mark Solms
Frankfurt a.M. December 2021

1 Introduction

On the dark side: chronic depression and trauma – signatures of our time? Some societal, conceptual and methodological considerations

Marianne Leuzinger-Bohleber

Hell

I am not alone with this loneliness
That is already one load less
And if I were to count us all
We were many …

Sometimes I had suicidal thoughts
And am not proud of it
Sometimes it seems like the only way out,
to silence them

All these thoughts make my life hell

In a live interview during the main French news (January 10, 2022, 20h) introducing the new album of the Belgian pop musician Stromae, the moderator asked the singer why he had disappeared from the public for seven years. Instead of responding verbally, Stromae sang his song "L'Enfer" directly into the camera. "By doing so he shook up not only the 7 million viewers, but countless more who watched the YouTube recordings afterwards. With his epochal high talent Stromae proved the ability of art to reach people inside" (Nils Minkmar in *Süddeutsche Zeitung*, 13.1.2022, p. 9).

The song hits a central feeling of life of many young people in these months of the pandemic, a feeling of life which they are sharing with chronically depressed patients, as will be discussed by many authors in this volume. As Stromae points out: he shares his suicidal pain and depression with many individuals in our Western societies. Depression has become a "Volkskrankheit" (illness of the people) in the 21st century, as I will discuss in the first paragraph of this introductory chapter (section 1). Clinical experiences as well as many large empirical studies have shown that psychoanalysis can help most of these depressed patients to find some light at the end of the tunnel of their psychic darkness due to a deep understanding of the many pathways which can lead into depression (cf. section 2). Moreover, many psychoanalysts were inspired by interdisciplinary knowledge

DOI: 10.4324/9781003279297-1

and research results from other disciplines (cf. section 3), although, historically, the relationship between psychoanalysis and academic research is a complex, tense issue (cf. section 4).[1]

1 Depression: a "Volkskrankheit" of the 21st century?

In recent decades depressions have increased to such an extent that, according to WHO estimates, depression will become the second most widespread disease worldwide in this decade (see e.g. Moussavi et al., 2007). For a long time depression was considered a disorder with a relatively good treatment prognosis, but this has changed in recent decades. Results from epidemiological research showed that depression is often a recurrent disorder with a high relapse rate and becomes chronic for 25–30% of those affected (see e.g. Steinert et al., 2014). There is also a high degree of comorbidity between depression and different personality disorders. In addition, pharmacological and short psychotherapeutic cognitive-behavioral as well as short psychotherapeutic treatment approaches have proved to be far less successful than hoped: 50% of depressed patients suffer a relapse after the first depressive episode, 70% after the second and 90% after the third episode; 50% of all depressed patients have a relapse after any form of short psychotherapy (see Blatt & Zuroff, 2005), 20–30% of all depressed patients do not respond positively to drugs at all (see e.g. Corveleyn, et al., 2013, Trivedi et al., 2011, Huhn et al., 2014). Of those with a positive response, one third has a relapse within one year, 75% within five years (see also Cuipers et al., 2017; Steinert et al., 2014). For these patients, long-term psychoanalytic therapies or psychoanalyses may offer an alternative (see Leichsenring 2008; Leichsenring & Rabung, 2011; Leuzinger-Bohleber et al., 2019, 2019a). In the representative DPV (Deutsche Psycho-analytische Vereinigung) outcome study, around 80% of all 402 former psycho-analysis patients or patients of long-term psychoanalytical therapies have shown sustained improvements in their psychopathological symptoms as well as in their object relations, professional quality and life quality. Among them were 27% who had been diagnosed as depressed mostly in combination with some personality disorders. To mention just one of the unexpected results of the study, 62% of the patients had been severely traumatized children of the Second World War (cf. Leuzinger-Bohleber et al., 2003).

Although depression can be regarded as one of the psychoanalytically best investigated disorders, the differentiation between its various forms is by no means easy and not yet sufficiently understood either in psychoanalytical or psychiatric terms. The older definition focused on psychogenic, endogenic and somatogenic depression, then DSM IV and ICD 10 started from the descriptive-symptomatic level and arrived at dimensionally different disorders (major depression, dysthymia, etc.). Without excluding the biological factors, in a psy-chodynamic understanding of depression the forms are not fanned out cate-gorically or dimensionally (see e.g. Hill, 2009, Hauser, 2008). Thus, as Sidney Blatt (2004) suggests, the different forms of depression can be located on a con-tinuum ranging from the dysphoric mood of microdepression to severe depression (see e.g. Fonagy & Luyten, 2009). Scarfone (Chapter 3 in this volume) writes on the fundamental differences between psychiatric and psychoanalytic diagnostical thinking:

> For us analysts, it matters that, contrary to diagnostic manuals such as the DSM, it is not so much the signs and symptoms – identified by the clinical *gaze* – but rather the challenge that these states pose to our *listening* that gives us the key to their differentiation. Psychoanalytic listening, in fact, helps us detect the specific metapsychological features of actual neuroses: from the *dynamic* point of view, the erasing of psychoneurotic conflictuality; from the *topical* point of view, the thinness if not the non-existence of the mediating function of the pre-conscious – namely a language without metaphors, without slips, without double meanings – and the impoverishment of the oneiric life; from the *economic* point of view, the tendency to motor discharge or else to a discharge that Freud called "secretory", that is to say, occurring inside the body, which contributes to somatizations. As Michel de M'Uzan indicated, even sexual activity in these cases takes on the value of a mere discharge of tension.[2] If we now look at the *temporal* point of view, we first notice a linearization of time, that is, the absence of the complex, *après-coup* time loops observable in psychoneurotic organizations. Moreover, in depression, time itself seems seriously slowed down if not arrested, sometimes fixated on opaque elements of previous history – something that often induces clinicians to invoke traumatic, organic or even genetic factors. The result of this arrested time is that the experience is always "present", or better: "actual", in the literal sense of Freud's adjective "*aktual*" in "*Aktualneurosen*" i.e. *presently active* with no apparent internal conflict or phantasmatic template. This means that the historical roots of the problem are not easily retrievable, and it is therefore difficult to relegate such "present" experience to the past. This makes me suggest that actual time, or the *unpast*, is the form of time pertaining to the dark core of psychic life.
>
> (Chapter 3, p. 6)

Scarfone describes two different poles in depression, melancholia and essential depression and illustrates this beautifully with a case example. Melancholia is a form of depression, as Freud described, as a psychic reaction to a (traumatic) loss of an object while essential depression can be seen as a result of real traumatization which is not mentally represented and thus can only be treated in highly frequent psychoanalyses. Christine Premmereur-Anzieu also discusses severe depressions caused on early trauma in her contribution in this volume:

> The blank depression in the mother and her psychic absence to which the patient as a child identified with, was the cause of an absence of representation: A void that doesn't allow for libidinal cathexis of a present object.
>
> (Chapter 12, p. 6)

According to Bohleber (2005, 2010), in *social sciences the depression has advanced to a signature of our time*, in which traditional structures and clear behavioral expectations have largely dissolved. Phenomena of delimitation and the enormous increase in individuals' choices of life perspectives result in a loss of social security and make one's own identity the lifelong project of the individual. In his study, the French sociologist Alain Ehrenberg (2016) declares the exhausted self to be the disease of contemporary society, whose behavioral norms are no longer based on guilt and discipline, but mainly on responsibility and initiative. The late bourgeois individual seems to be replaced by an individual who has the idea that "everything is possible" and is marked by fear for his self-realization, which can easily increase to the feeling of exhaustion. The pressure for individualization is reflected in feelings of failure, shame and insufficiency and finally in depressive symptoms. For Ehrenberg, if neurosis is the illness of the individual torn apart by the conflict between what is allowed and what is forbidden, depression is the illness of the individual inhibited and exhausted by the tension between what is possible and what is impossible. Depression thus becomes a tragedy of inadequacy (for the role of social and cultural factors in depression, see e.g. Jiménez, 2019, Jiménez, Botto & Fonagy, 2021).

Such epistemological–clinical data and social–scientific analyses also challenge psychoanalysis to re-examine the issue of depression and evaluate the state of its research. Therefore, in 2004, a multi-center research group of psychoanalysts and cognitive behaviorists decided to initiate a comparative psychotherapy study on the outcomes of cognitive-behavioral and psychoanalytic long-term treatments, the so-called *LAC study*. We conceptualized the study in close collaboration with the research group of Phil Richardson, Peter Fonagy and David Taylor who also – at that time – planned a study on the outcome of long-term psychoanalytic psychotherapies in difficult-to-treat depression, the so-called *Tavistock-Depression Study*. We used a number of identical measuring instruments to compare the data from the two studies. Close collaboration was also established on the psychoanalytic conceptualization of depression. David Taylor had just written first versions of the Tavistock Treatment Manual for the treatment of difficult-to-treat depressive patients. He agreed to train the psychoanalytic study therapists of the LAC study, a prerequisite for us to include psychoanalysts of various psychoanalytical orientations as study therapists.[3]

In the meantime both the results of the Tavistock study (Fonagy, Rost et al., 2015) and the LAC study (Leuzinger-Bohleber et al., 2019, 2019a) have been published. These and several other studies show the positive outcomes of long-term psychoanalytic therapies for depressed patients. However, the problem remains: most outcome studies to date have focused on short-term therapies. The outcomes of psychoanalytic short-term therapies according to evidence-based medicine criteria have meanwhile been confirmed by many studies (see e.g. Fonagy, 2015; Shedler, 2010, 2015, Abbass et al., 2009, Driessen et al., 2010, De Maat et al., 2013, Kächele & Thomä, 2000; Kächele et al., 2006). Liliengren

(2019) has collected 272 RCT studies in this field until now (see also the third edition of the *Open-Door Review*, Leuzinger-Bohleber, Arnold & Kächele, 2015/ 2019). In contrast, still only a few studies are available on the effects of long-term psychotherapies and psychoanalyses (see e.g. Blomberg, 2001; Sandell et al., 2001; Grande et al., 2009; Huber & Klug, 2016; Knekt et al., 2011; Fonagy, Rost et al., 2015; Leichsening, 2008, Leichsening & Rabung, 2011). This is one of the main reasons for planning a kind of a replication study of the LAC Study: the *Multi-Level Outcome Study of Psychoanalyses of Chronically Depressed Patients with Early Trauma (MODE)*. It follows on from the results of the *LAC Depression Study*, which showed that chronically depressed patients can be successfully treated with psychoanalytic (PAT) and cognitive-behavioral long-term therapy (CBT) (high effect sizes in symptom reduction, high remission rates etc.). It was found that structural changes (measured with Operationalized Psychodynamic Diagnostics, OPD) can only be observed in PAT but not in CBT after three years of treatment. One unexpected result of the LAC study was that around 80% of chronic depressives suffered from early trauma and responded particularly well to high frequency psychoanalyses (see also Negele et al., 2015). One of MODE's aims is to investigate this group of difficult-to-treat patients. In other words: the study focuses on the question whether there are certain patient groups that require intensive long-term treatments in order to achieve sustained improvements in their chronic depression. In addition, it will be investigated whether and how symptomatic and structural changes in this patient group can also be investigated with neurobiological instruments. For this reason, MODE considers neurobiological (e.g. fMRI) and clinical–psychoanalytical (e.g. changes in dreams) observation methods in addition to the usual (psychological) instruments of comparative psychotherapy research (see Ambresin, Fischmann & Leuzinger-Bohleber, Chapter 13 in this volume, Fischmann, Leuzinger-Bohleber & Ambresin, Chapter 14 in this volume, Moser & von Zeppelin, 1996; Peterson et al., 2019.

The following introduction is based on a Workbook (treatment manual) which was written with the aim of training the study therapists of MODE (Leuzinger-Bohleber, Fischmann & Beutel, in press). It is based on the rich clinical experiences of psychoanalytical long-term treatments in the LAC Study. Furthermore the knowledge of some central papers conceptualizing psychoanalytic treatments of chronic depressed patients with early traumatizations are integrated (Taylor, 2010; Bleichmar, 1996, 2010; Bohleber & Leuzinger-Bohleber, 2016; Lane et al., 2015), as well as other contemporary psychoanalytic and interdisciplinary knowledge on depression and trauma.

As is well known, knowledge gained in these intensive, long-term psychoanalytic treatments still forms the basis for many applications in short psychodynamic and psychoanalytical interventions in different psychiatric and psychological settings, e.g. crisis interventions, various forms of short therapies (e.g. the transference focused psychotherapy (TFP) of the group around Kernberg and Clarkin (cf. Caligor et al., 2018), mentalized based treatment (MBT) by Fonagy et al. (cf. Fonagy & Luyten, 2009), focal therapies (cf.

Leuzinger-Bohleber et al., 2019)) or different forms of psychoanalytical group or family therapies, to name but a few. In the limited context of this introduction, the psychoanalytical knowledge of the psychodynamics of depression is first briefly summarized in today's psychoanalysis and some of the important historical lines are outlined (section 2). In section 3 this knowledge is compared with selected interdisciplinary findings on trauma and depression from the field of Embodied Cognitive Science and neuroscientific memory research. A first attempt at integration of psychoanalytical and interdisciplinary knowledge is discussed.

2 Some basic lines of a psychoanalytic understanding of depression

In this section I will summarize the major findings of conceptual and clinical psychoanalytical research on depression relatively shortly because I assume that most of this knowledge is well known in the meantime.

2.1 Depression as a reaction to loss, guilt and reparation

In contemporary psychoanalysis depression is still seen as the reaction to a loss, that of a real object in the outside reality of the patient or that of an inner object, a loss of an internal relationship. The focus of the psychoanalytic investigation, however, is not the object loss itself, but its mental processing. In "Mourning and Melancholia" (1917) Sigmund Freud distinguishes mourning from melancholia. Mourning is a feeling "out of tune" with a painful mood, a suspension of interest in the outside world, the loss of the ability to love, and an inhibition of creativity in work and one's leisure time. All this serves the devotion to mourning and the facilitation of mourning work ("Trauerarbeit"). The mourning individual painfully works through their memories of the lost object in order to be able to remove the libidinal cathexis from the object and finally to accept the loss. If the withdrawal of the libido is successful, then the grief comes to an end and the ego is "free and uninhibited again". Metaphorically speaking: the libido can now look for other objects. The pathological sadness of melancholia may be complicated by the fact that an already existing deep ambivalence towards the object has been intensified by narcissistic insults, setbacks and disappointments on the part of the object. In contrast to normal grief, the object cannot be abandoned, the attachment is preserved by being incorporated into the ego through narcissistic identification. Now the ego feels the hatred that originally was directed towards the object, the ego is insulted, denigrated and humiliated. The love relationship has been taken back to the level of sadism. But at the same time the process of identification establishes a "critical voice" in the ego. The object chosen according to the narcissistic type assumes the role of a kind of judge as (unconscious) part of the ego, and the accusations against the object become self-reproaches. One of Freud's most important insights into melancholia was the discovery of the development of the individual subject, as he formulated it in 1923 in "The Ego and the Id". The replacement of the cathexis of the object by identification becomes its constituent condition. The character of the ego is now formed by the "permanent traces of old object relations". Thus Freud also revises his strict separation between mourning and melancholia because early object relationships always shape the personality structure of the self, thanks to the continuous identification with them.

Accordingly, the cathexis (and the attachment) of the lost object is not simply abandoned, but transformed in a restructuring process, whereby the memories can become a permanent component of the inner world (Hagmann 1995): with structural theory and his insights into the influence of the superego, Freud can better grasp the conflicts and tensions between the superego and the ego. The overpowering superego seizes the consciousness of the depressive and rages against the ego. It has seized the sadism of the individual and turned it destructively against the ego. Freud now calls this mental constellation prevailing in the superego a "pure culture of the death instinct", which often enough succeeds in actually driving the ego to death.

Karl Abraham had already identified hatred as the cause of depression in 1911, which led to repressed self-accusations and feelings of guilt. In 1924, like Freud, he also recognized identification as a fundamental mechanism. If the person predisposed to depression loses his love object, he reacts with hatred and contempt, the frustrating object is ejected and, in the course of regression to the oral-sadistic stage, is immediately introjected back into the self. Through this narcissistic identification with the devalued object, the ego itself becomes worthless and reacts melancholically.

This psychodynamic understanding of depression described by Freud and Abraham has been taken up by various psychoanalytic researchers. The decisive determinant for the outbreak of depression is not the loss of the real object itself, but a constitutional heightening of ambivalence or aggression that intensifies it, which originates from narcissistic offenses by and disappointments in the object. Sándor Radó, Melanie Klein and Edith Jacobson further explored the sadistic aggressiveness of the superego as one important factor of depression. In Melanie Klein's work, the archaic severity of the early super-ego comes from the splitting of the object- and self-representations into an "ideal good object" on the one hand and a "fantasized evil one" on the other hand. Through the later integration of these splits in the representations the child becomes aware of their own aggression against the idealized primary object and falls into a depression. Melanie Klein introduces the new concept of reparation in the so-called depressive position. Depression occurs when the libidinal and aggressive impulses, thoughts and drives can be integrated and reparation associated with it can be achieved. If excessive aggressive impulses are dominating the libidinal ones, such an integration and reparation cannot take place: a depression develops.[4]

Edith Jacobson describes a basic conflict that can be found in all depressive states. If the ego cannot achieve the satisfaction it desires and cannot use its aggression for achieving this satisfaction, then it turns the aggressive impulses against the self-representation. A narcissistic conflict develops between the desired self-image and the image of the failing devalued self. The self-esteem is lost and a depressive mood develops. Severe depressions are found above all in people whose early frustrations and disappointments had such devastating effects because they reacted with unusual hostility. Early frustrations create excessive expectations, love objects are idealized, ego ideals and desire-determined self-images are exaggerated and unattainable. New narcissistic insults lead to a devaluation of the love object. In order to endure these insults and make up for them, glorified grandiosity fantasies of the love objects are introjected into the superego; the devalued fantasies of a bad parent, on the other hand, are introjected into the ego. Thus the child can hold on to the hope of love in the future, but from now on is exposed to the massive criticism and hostility of these idealized unconscious fantasies and representations. At the same time the narcissistic self-regulation of the ego is damaged.

2.2 Narcissistic and psychotic depression

Psychoanalytical authors have repeatedly addressed the fact that in depressive patients the ego is particularly vulnerable and intolerant of frustration and disappointment. Also, self-representations and object representations do not yet seem to be sufficiently differentiated from each other. In 1927, Sándor Radó had already noticed the special tendency of depressive patients to adopt passive–dependent object relationships, because this was the only way they could maintain their self-esteem. A somewhat different basic understanding of depressive basic conflicts now follows on from this. It places the basic disorder in the narcissistic regulatory system and describes it as the tension between strongly pronounced narcissistic expectations and ideals on the one hand and the inability to meet these ideals or to receive narcissistic support from the object for them on the other. This then results in the depressive affect. In 1952, Eduard Bibring was the first to elaborate on this explanatory approach and to separate it from the assumption of aggression directed at the self as the main determining factor of depression. Depression is "an emotional expression of a state of helplessness of the self". It is a mode of reaction generally available to humans. The ego often finds itself in a state of real or imaginary helplessness in the face of overwhelming difficulties. Others speak of *narcissistic depression*, given the underlying tensions between ego and ego ideal. The dominant feelings here are not feelings of guilt fed by aggression and self-hatred, but shame and humiliation and feelings of abandonment and helplessness. In 1965 Sandler and Joffe describe the loss of narcissistic integrity as the central cause of the depressive affective reaction. It is not so much the loss of a love object that is in the foreground as the loss of the well-being that is inseparably linked to it. It is a feeling of having been deprived of an ideal state of the mind. If the individual feels helpless and resigned in the face of the mental pain experienced and cannot resort to an outwardly directed aggression to remedy it, he or she reacts affectively with a depression. Wolfgang Loch (1967) also assumes an imbalance between the ideals of the individuals and their self-esteem. The perception of this discrepancy produces the depressive affect. In the depressive patient there is no stable connection between the self and the ideal-self, because the process of identifying the self with the ideal-object is disturbed by aggressive impulses and attitudes. Thus the connection between self and ideal-self is only guaranteed as long as the real presence of an ideal-object is given. In *psychotic depression*, the ideal-self is lost, forcing the cathexis of the superego as a substitute. This archaic–persecutory superego has taken the consciousness function of the ego and robbed the depressive of his self-esteem: the real self-assessment gets lost. Because the libidinal cathexis of the ideal object was already disturbed in early childhood, depressive feeling of emptiness and inhibition of vitality develop later in life.

2.3 Integrative models of depression

Another group of psychoanalysts does not attempt to describe one central basic conflict, but rather to develop an integrative model of depressive states of mind in view of the diversity of pathogenic conflict constellations in depression. Stavros Mentzos (1995) starts from narcissistic self-regulation, which is carried by a mature ideal-self, ideal-object and superego in a mature self-regulation. A blocking or pathological development of one of these factors of the self-regulation leads to different clinical pictures of depression (e.g. mania, anaclitic depression and guilt depression). Herbert Will (1994) orders the different types of depression on the basis of leading emotions: superego or guilt depression with guilt and self-accusation; oral-dependent depression with anxious longing and disappointment; ego depression with helplessness and hopelessness; narcissistic depression with shame and self-denigration.

Based on many empirical studies, Sidney J. Blatt (2004) characterized two different organizations of depression: the anaclitic type, which centers around interpersonal factors such as dependence, helplessness, feelings of loss and abandonment. In contrast: the introjective type shows a strict, punitive superego, self-criticism, low self-esteem, basic feelings of failure and guilt.

Bleichmar (1996) attributes a major role in the outbreak of depression to the feeling of helplessness and hopelessness. In the predepressive individual there is fixation on a desire that occupies a central position in the libidinal economy of the subject and cannot be replaced by any other. This desire appears to be unattainable, leading to a sense of deep helplessness and a self-representation of powerlessness. A feeling of hopelessness spreads, which extends not only to the present, but also to the future. They lead to an increasing deactivation of the efforts to still fulfill the wish, and depressive affects, apathy and psychomotor inhibition are the result. There are various different pathways that cause a depressive state and determine it. None is obligatory, each is determined by different factors and psychodynamic constellations. As discussed in section 2.1, most authors give aggression a prominent or even universal place in the determination of depression (see dynamics on the upper left part of Figure 1.1). In addition to this, Bleichmar lists the following factors: guilt and feelings of guilt;

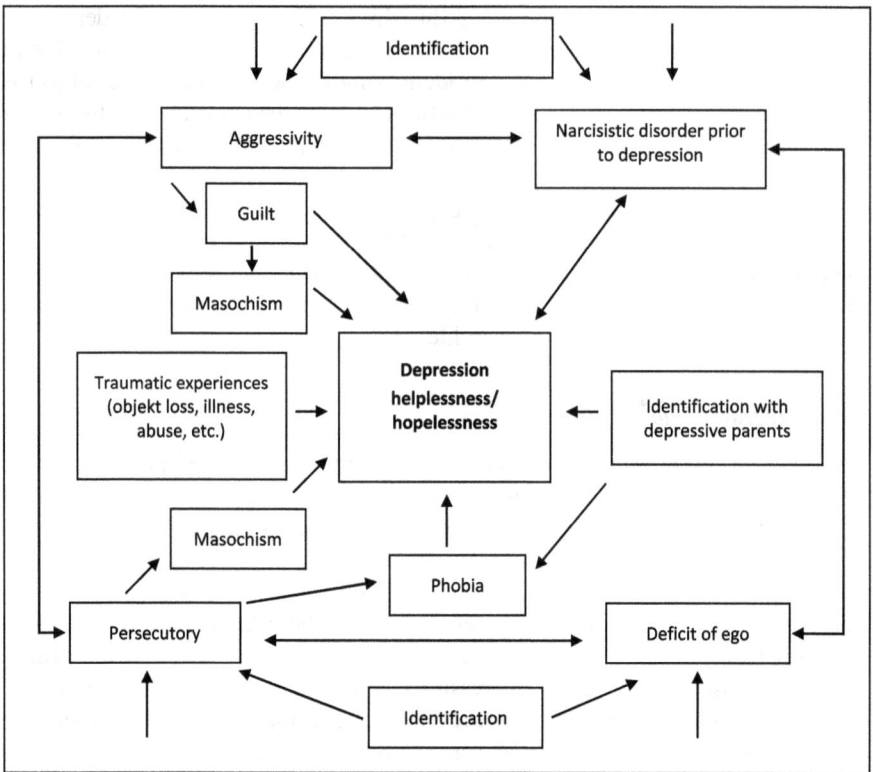

Figure 1.1 Pathways to depression (Bleichmar, 1996).

frustration in the realization of narcissistic aspirations; narcissistic personality disorders (either with weak narcissistic self-regulation or with traits of grandiosity and omnipotence collapsing through reality; dynamics on the upper left side of Figure 1.1); persecution fears; ego deficits; traumatic experiences. These factors can be effective individually, but also in combination or in succession, as Bleichmar (1996) illustrates in Figure 1.1 with three extended case examples.

Siri Gullestad, in her contribution in this volume (Chapter 17), adds some additional causal factors leading into depression to the different pathways described by Bleichmar:

> Furthermore, psychoanalysis underlines the significance of needs that are not represented in words (Gullestad, 2003). Loss may occur at a stage of development where a mental representation of a specific object has not yet been established ("la chose", Kristeva, 1987). We are here dealing with a specific modality of depression, "le deuil blanc" (Green, 1983) characterised by *le négatif* – i.e. absence, emptiness. Mourning is made difficult because affects are invested in "la chose" – the thing beyond words.

3 Depression and trauma: some interdisciplinary findings

3.1 Depression and embodied memories of trauma[5]

The extreme feeling of helplessness and hopelessness is not only, as just outlined, a central basic feeling of depression, but also characterizes the traumatic experience. As Bohleber (2010, 2012) points out, the traumatic situation can result in an extreme sense of helplessness, linked to the overwhelming anxiety often confronted with the danger of death or annihilation as well as an experience of being completely left alone:

> Psychoanalytic trauma theories have evolved on the basis of two models, one psycho-economic, the other hermeneutic and based on object relations theory. In order to grasp the phenomenology and long-term consequences of trauma, we need both models. The psycho-economical model focuses on excessive arousal and on anxiety that cannot be contained by the psyche and that breaks through the shield against stimuli. The model based on object relations focuses on the breakdown of internal communication which produces an experience of total abandonment, precluding the integration of trauma by narrative means.
>
> (Bohleber 2010, 2012, p. xxi; see also Cooper, 1986, p. 44, Leuzinger-
> Bohleber, 2015)

The traumatic experience breaks down both the basic trust of the traumatized individual in a helping object (see Erikson, 1958/1993, see also the concept of epistemic trust by Fonagy, Luyten & Allison, 2015) on the one hand and the basic trust in one's own self-agency on the other hand (see e.g. Emde & Leuzinger-Bohleber, 2014; Leuzinger-Bohleber, 2015). The traumatized person is unconsciously and firmly convinced that nobody can help them in a situation of extreme, life threatening danger and dehumanization, and that they are totally left alone and completely incapable of freeing themself from the unbearable situation.

The psychoanalytic knowledge of short-term and long-term effects of extreme traumatization is mainly based on clinical psychoanalytical experiences with survivors of the Shoa and their children and grandchildren. The kinds of experiences that the victims of the Shoa went through exceeds our imagination. The incomprehensibility of the trauma is described in psychoanalytic–scientific general concepts like extreme traumatization (cf., e.g.

Krystal, 1968/2015) or sequential (Keilson, 1991) or cumulative traumatizations (Khan, 1964). The survivors of such extreme traumatizations illustrated that such traumatizations are not processed psychically, but lead to lifelong disturbances such as nightmares, flashbacks, loneliness and depression, dissociation and derealization, disturbances in the sense of time and basic feeling of identity, diffuse panic, fear and aggression attacks, emotional encapsulations, breakdown of basic trust in a helping Other and self-agency (see above), as well as the basic meanings of life. Some of the psychosomatic symptoms include sleep disturbances, bodily pain that is not easy to localize, etc. The suffering linked to these deep psychic wounds can be relieved in long psychotherapy, but the wounds can never really be (fully) "healed". Besides, the experienced trauma is often transmitted to the second and third generation.

For comprehensible reasons it took nearly 60 years until psychoanalysts in Germany started to talk about the effects of severe traumatization on the families of the persecutors and by-standers during the time of National socialism. The concern about equating the horrifying singularity of the Shoah with the families who had been actively involved in Nazi crimes is still justified. Regardless, German psychoanalysts tried to make sense of the unexpected results of the DPV Follow-Up Study mentioned above: around 62% of the 402 patients who underwent psychoanalysis during the 1980s had been traumatized as former children of the war (see e.g. Leuzinger-Bohleber et al. 2003; Radebold, Heuft & Fooken, 2006). Additionally, as already mentioned above, one unexpected finding of the LAC depression study was that 84% of the chronically depressed patents had gone through severe childhood trauma (Negele et al., 2015). To cut a long story short: psychoanalysts in Germany (as well as in other European countries) are treating many traumatized patients due to the long (mainly unconscious) shadows of the extreme man-made-disasters of the Second World War and the Nationalsozialism on the second and third generations. They are still living in traumatized societies!

Hence, many clinical and empirical studies show the short-term and long-term consequences of traumatization due to so-called man-made-disasters. The traumatic experiences lead to great vulnerability of the traumatized after the escape from acute danger (cf. in addition among other things, Bohleber 2010, 2012; see e.g. Laub, 2005; Bodenstab, 2015). This vulnerability makes them hypersensitive especially to human relationships in general and, of course, also to the therapeutic relationship. I have discussed some of the consequences of these findings for the treatment techniques of chronically depressed, early traumatized patients in some extended case studies (e.g. Leuzinger-Bohleber, 2015a).

As Bohleber & Leuzinger-Bohleber (2016) discussed, in many cases traumatic experiences can only be fragmentarily recollected because they are dissociated entirely from current consciousness. In psychoanalysis or psychoanalytic therapy, they repeat themselves in enactments and other manifestations in the transference.

Generations of psychoanalysts since Freud have concerned themselves with the way in which repetition in transference can be rendered a healing process of remembering. This primarily involves symbolically represented and repressed memories or relationship patterns. However, theory and clinical psychoanalysis has focused for quite some time on psychic material present in the analytical relationship in other, *not yet symbolized, "unrepresented" ways*. Levine, Reed and Scarfone entitled their anthology "Unrepresented States and the Construction of Meaning" (2013, in honor of André Green), and focus on the question of the search for meaning in the unrepresented from a contemporary perspective. With his broadly received concept of "dead mother", Green (2007) described the early identification with an absent mother leading to a withdrawal cathexis and thus to a disappearance of the inner representation which, in the transference relationship, can be perceived by the analyst as an empty, negative hallucination of the object, "a representation of the absence of representation" (Green, 1999c, p. 196, quoted in Reed, 2013, p. 39). Reed (2013, p. 29 ff.) points out that this negative hallucination of the object leads to an emptiness rather than a representation of the lost object – an empty mirror, which, with these patients is always there, but which is frequently observed in the analysand's extreme reactions to separation from the analyst. Green is concerned with the process of de-objectification, namely, the obliteration of representation. Other psychoanalysts, by contrast, focused on the psychic material of patients, which had only insufficiently, if at all, gone through the processes of symbolization. Dominique Scarfone (2013) presented a conceptual integration of different forms of psychic representation and their various psychoanalytic conceptualizations. He compared Pierce's sign theory to Freud's conception of primary and secondary processes, Lacan's theory of the real, the imaginary and the symbolic, Wilfred Bion's beta and alpha elements, Jean Laplanche's infantile sexual theories and their decoding in analytic discourse, and Pierra Aulangier's concept of the primary, such as "primary violence", which entered the stage ("mis-en-scène") and could ultimately open up the discourse on secondary processes: a brilliant example of contemporary concept research.

In many papers Leuzinger-Bohleber and Pfeifer (e.g. 2002) pursued another path by drawing on several studies in the field of basic research, more specifically, Embodied Cognitive Science and the Cognitive Neurosciences, so as to show that these disciplines offer first explanations for the clinically important phenomenon, such as the analyst's spontaneous inspiration, their associations to the "unrepresented" which can be an initial central step to understanding hitherto unrepresented psychic material, and which is capable of making psychoanalytic processing accessible at all (see also Vivona, 2009). Hence, this should provide new perspectives on familiar concepts, such as "scenic understanding" (Argelander, Lorenzer), "hearing with the third ear" (Reik), "cracking up" (Bollas) or the "now-moments" by the *Boston Change Process Study Group*. Furthermore, aspects of current discourse on intersubjective psychoanalysis and on enactment are touched on, as well as further understanding of countertransference around the bodily sensations of the analyst. Their considerations can also be related to works on musicality, dynamically emotional syntax and performance of the analytic relationship (cf., among others, Gaensbauer, 2011; Knox, 2009; Marshall, 2009; Leuzinger-Bohleber, 2015).

Inspired by biology and the life sciences, Embodied Cognitive Science currently understands memory not as a retrieval of stored knowledge in the brain but as a function of the entire organism, the product of complex, dynamic recategorization and interactive processes that are always embodied (cf. among others, Edelman, 1987; 1989; Lakoff & Johnson, 1999; Damasio, 1994; Pfeifer and Bongard, 2007; Leuzinger-Bohleber and Pfeifer, 2002, Leuzinger-Bohleber, 2015). The human organism – and the human psyche – is in an ongoing (embodied) state of transformation involved in constant dynamic processes of interaction with the environment in which a continuous process of recategorizing experiences occurs. Memories of earlier situations unconsciously determine present thought, feelings and action, though not in the sense of stored knowledge in analogy to a computer or static memory traces. In contrast, memories are products of dynamic, complex constructions in the here and now. In the sense of embodiment, sensorimotor coordinations in the present always operate in an analogue manner as was the case in earlier situations. The similarities between a current and a past situation are not perceived cognitively, e.g. by cognitive pattern matching, but by similar complex information gained by different senses (auditory, visual, olfactory, touch, smell etc.) and actions of the body (characterized as sensorimotor coordination in Embodied Cognitive Science). Through such sensorimotor coordination, memories and categories are constructed automatically as a self-regulating process of learning by doing (John Dewey), in other words, by means through coordinating information from sensory channels and connected (motor) actions of the body. Memories resulting from sensorimotor coordination thus provide orientation in a new situation.

A brief example may illustrate the processes of building categories involved in learning by doing. If you put a bar of chocolate in one hand of a one-year-old boy and a bar of colored wood in the other, the child will immediately put both bars in his mouth. Only a very few trials are required before he prefers the chocolate: through sensorimotor coordination, he has developed the categories "chocolate" and "wooden bar" without having the categories explained to him, but solely through learning by doing, by sensorimotor coordination.

Another field of research is important for understanding social interaction in general, and transference relationships in particular. Recent studies have illustrated the decisive role of the so-called mirror neuron system, which enables human beings to identify immediately with the observed behavior and the mental state of others (see, for instance, Gallese, 2009, 2013; Shapiro, 2009). In the psychoanalytic treatment, this means that during interaction with the analysand, analogue sensorimotor coordinations take place within the psychoanalyst, as in the analysand implying that unconscious processes of immediate identifications are occurring. These processes bring forth categories of understanding – automatically, spontaneously and unconsciously – which are connected with the analysand's unconsciously occurring memory processes from earlier, important relationship experiences. In the case of traumatized patients these are recurring memories of psychically and physiologically unbearable experiences of flooding stimuli, of extreme powerlessness, desperation, pain, of panic and fear of death. By identifying with the analysand's ongoing sensorimotor coordination and the construction of memories of the traumatic experiences in his countertransference, the psychoanalyst immediately (unconsciously) understands the traumatic psychic reality of the patient. And yet, at the same time, the extreme quality of traumatic experiences mobilize his own spontaneous defense, thereby hindering becoming conscious of what he has unconsciously perceived in the interaction with his analysand. Christine Premmereur-Anzieu, coming from a different psychoanalytical background, describes similar psychoanalytical tasks with early traumatized, chronically depressed individuals in her contribution in this volume (Chapter 12). "The patient, who cannot express with words the neglects or failures of the early environment, will signify the defect and its consequences through the body. By echoing the patient archaic experiences, the analyst gives a circular relation where the perceptions and sensations are shared, contained and expressed through words" (p. 114, see also her case example, illustrating this technique of the analyst; see also the case example in Chapter 3 by Dominique Scarfone in this volume).

To summarize: formerly, memories have been explained by way of a model of representation in which, due to excessive arousal, traumatic experiences are not psychically integrated, but incompletely represented or not even registered. Contemporary interdisciplinary research results are now available following radical rethinking on the conception of memory and recollection which are changing the understanding of memories and their relevance for transformation processes in psychoanalysis. This new interdisciplinary knowledge has consequences for the treatment technique of chronically depressed, early traumatized patients, which we have so frequently treated in the LAC study (see Bohleber & Leuzinger-Bohleber, 2016, Leuzinger-Bohleber, 2008, 2012, 2015, Scarfone, Chapter 3 in this volume).

3.2 Trauma, depression and memory consolidation

Lane et al. (2015), in their introduction to an important review of current memory research and its implications for various psychotherapies in the journal *Brain and Behavioral Sciences*, refer to the beginnings of psychoanalysis as a trauma theory. Freud and Breuer (see Freud, 1895) postulated in their first theory that the child's inability to express emotions during the trauma of sexual seduction is the cause of hysterical disease and must therefore be "dissipated" in catharsis. As we know, this thesis proved to be too simplified: the oedipal fantasies replaced the real, traumatic experience. The re-experience of early childhood conflicts and fantasies in the transference and their elaboration in the analytical relationship took their place. As Bohleber (2010; 2012) pointed out, the consequences of early childhood traumatizations in psychoanalysis then receded into the background and, especially in their implications for treatment techniques, were even neglected for a long time (see above).

According to Lane et al. (2015, p. 3 ff), a large number of neurobiological studies on trauma confirm the concept of the dynamic unconscious of psychoanalysis in a new way. Traumatizations are preserved in the unconscious because of their emotionally overwhelming quality, but, metaphorically speaking, they continue to have an effect and determine inadequate pathological thinking, feeling and action in our patients. Another agreement of the authors with psychoanalytical approaches is that they postulate that the traumatic, emotionally unbearable experience in the therapeutic relationship must be revived – in all forms of psychotherapy – if these lead to real, lasting changes. The research group around Lane et al. (2015) justify this thesis with the concept of memory consolidation.

> In this paper, we propose that change occurs by activating old memories and their associated emotions, and introducing new emotional experiences in therapy enabling new emotional elements to be incorporated into that memory trace via reconsolidation. Moreover, change will be enduring to the extent that this reconsolidation process occurs in a wide variety of environmental settings and contents. This proposed mechanism may be timely … We propose an integrated memory model with three associative components – autobiographical (event) memories, semantic structures, and emotional responses – that are inextricably linked and that, combined, lead to maladaptive behaviors.
>
> (p. 3)

Through the therapeutic activation of old memories and emotional reactions associated with them, new traces of memory are created that also modify the old, "pathological" ones. The corrective relationship experience takes place in a new context, the therapeutic setting itself (i.e. in the transference relationship), which is associated with the old memory, namely through the process of reactivation, re-encoding and re-consolidation (see Ryan et al., 2008). Through the "updating" of memories of earlier events through new experiences, the associated knowledge, rules and schemata are also changed. Therefore, new semantic structures, rules and schemes are developed that, through therapeutic processing, can lead to a more adequate way of interpreting events and linking them to more appropriate emotional responses. These changes are sustainable if they lead to re-consolidation processes in different contexts, leading to a generalization of the newly developed memory structures and their semantic contents to new situations and environments (see Lane et al. 2015, p. 3).

Lane summarizes two different theories of memory consolidation: the "standard model of memory consolidation" (Squire & Alvarez, 1995) emphasizes that the structures of the brain change from the medial temporal lobe (including the hippocampus) to neocortical structures including the prefrontal cortex. It is important that the content of the memory remains unchanged through this consolidation process. Nadel and Moscovitch (1997) developed an alternative theory of memory consolidation, the so-called multiple trace theory (MTT). Instead of focusing primarily on the time course of memory consolidation, the theory deals with the question of how repeated memories of earlier events lead to a strengthening of the memory representation of the original event. Analogous to the "standard model of consolidation", the MTT postulates that the development of long-term memories requires a permanent interaction between the hippocampal region of the medial temporal lobe and the neocortical regions. But in contrast to standard theory, MTT postulates that the hippocampal region remains an integral part of memory traces and is therefore always involved when episodic memories are retrieved from long-term memory, no matter how old these memories may be. The evidence for this theory comes from fMRI studies. The classical theory assumes a phase of instability immediately after the event, which is successively replaced by a stabilization of memory in which the memories can no longer be changed. MTT theory, on the other hand, postulates a much more dynamic understanding of memory, which coincides with the psychoanalytical concept of "Nachträglichkeit".

According to MTT, the old memory contents and the emotions associated with them are therefore activated with each new memory, but they change each time anew – due to the current context of the processing – and thus acquire, as the concept of "Nachträglichkeit" (Freud) describes, a current, "new" meaning; this, as Freud explains in the case of "Emma", can ascribe a traumatic quality to earlier experiences, even through development-specific (adolescent) conflicts and fantasies.

Interestingly, the research group refers in its arguments to the "false memory debate" of the 1990s and the many empirical studies which show that memories are constantly rewritten and therefore never depict the "historical truth" in a "one-to-one" sense. They adapt in a flexible way to the narrative context in which they are told. It is precisely this phenomenon that Lane et al. (2015) use as an argument for why the new, reliable, professional relationship experiences in psychotherapy hold the chance to change unbearable emotions that have not yet been psychologically integrated, which go hand in hand with the corresponding (implicit) memories and irrational convictions: since memories are "adaptive", they can use the security of the new relationship experience to adapt inadequate emotions and convictions anew and more adequately to the here and now.

Lane et al. (2015) then investigate the different roles implicit emotions play in different psychotherapies: in behavioral therapy, in cognitive-behavioral therapy, in emotion-focused therapy (EFT, a further development of Roger's non directive psychotherapy) and in psychoanalysis. Since emotional reactions, as well as episodic and semantic memory, do not function independently of each other, as was long assumed, but interact with each other in a more complex way, memory structures can use "different entrance gates" in the integrative memory model outlined by Lane et al. (2015) in Figure 1.2.

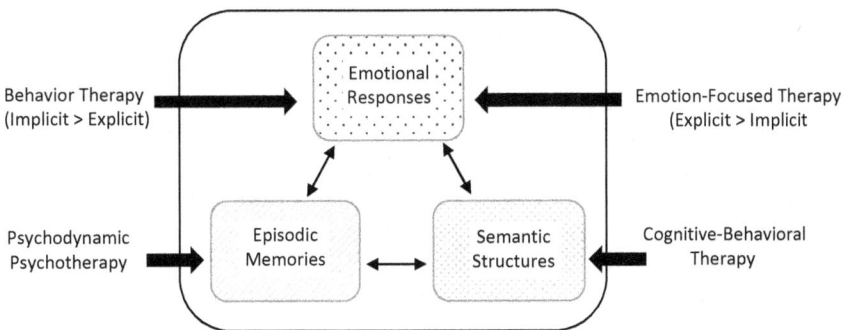

Figure 1.2 Integrative memory model (Lane et al. 2015).

"Classical behavioral therapy" (BT), which has proved successful in many studies such as in the treatment of patients with post-traumatic stress disorder, tries, e.g. in exposure therapy, to make inadequate emotions, which are implicitly connected with traumatization, explicit in a safe therapeutic relationship and thus not to "extinguish" them but to change them or adapt them to the current environment (environmental contingencies). According to Lane et al. (2015), BT is therefore suitable for the treatment of patients with disorders in specific, identifiable situations with implicit, inadequate emotions, such as patients with phobias.

Cognitive-behavioral therapy (CBT) starts with pathological beliefs (irrational thoughts) (i.e. semantic memory structures) associated with traumatic emotions and attempts to correct them through psychoeducation, exercises and homework, i.e. to change the semantic memory.

Emotion-focused therapy (EPF), as mentioned above, a further development of Roger's non directive psychotherapy and Gestalt therapy, aims to change emotions through emotions. Analogous to a focused transfer concept (e.g. in psychoanalytic focal therapy or crisis interventions), EPF therapists try to activate the unbearable emotions associated with traumatic experiences directly in the therapeutic relationship and to associate them with alternative, corrective emotions. Explicit emotional reactions in therapy are associated with the implicit, the original traumatic experience. According to Lane, both CBT and EPF are suitable for treating patients with symptomatic syndromes such as depression who are not situation-specific but have temporary disorders in explicit emotional behavior.

In contrast, there is a differential indication for psychoanalytic psychotherapies in patients with character pathologies that are not situation-specific and temporary, in other word, patients with chronic diseases, because psychoanalytic treatments offer the advantage that they examine early unconscious pathological object relation experiences which have entered, e.g. into the procedural memory, directly in the transference relationship.

> Time and cost considerations aside, the technique of meeting three, four or five times per week for several years creates a special opportunity to activate old memories and observe their influence on present-day construal and emotional experiences with an emotional intensity and vividness that is difficult or impossible with other methods (Freud 1914/1958). As such, this approach has the potential to offer something not available with other modalities that can have pervasive effects on a person's functioning in a wide variety of social, occupational, and avocational settings. New learning can involve improvement in function above and beyond symptom reduction, such as better self-esteem, greater ability to tolerate and manage stress, improved flexibility in social relations, a greater capacity for intimacy and the construction of a coherent life narrative that exceeds what would be expected based on symptomatic improvement alone (Shedler, 2010).
>
> (Lane et al., 2015, p. 16)

In the MODE study mentioned above, we take up this hypothesis of Lane et al. (2015) and test it empirically (see Ambresin, Fischmann and Leuzinger-Bohleber, Chapter 13 in this volume; Peterson et al. 2019).

4 Some historical remarks on research in psychoanalysis

As is well known, the question of what kind of science psychoanalysis is has shaped our discipline from the beginning. George Makari (2008) impressively traces back the origins of psychoanalysis to the beginning of the 20th century and shows how much it is the product of European cultural and intellectual history. In his understanding of psychoanalysis, Freud succeeded in integrating various currents of biology, physiology, psychophysics and psychology at the time. For instance the controversies surrounding a new understanding of psychopathology around Charcot at the world-famous Salpetière Clinic in France, as well as the scientific study of human sexuality by Krafft-Ebing, Ehrenfels, Weinberger, Moll, Hirschfeld and others influenced Freud's theories of psychosexual development, the unconscious and the psychodynamics of mental disorders (see Makari, 2008, p. 120). Moreover, in this scientific orientation Freud was strongly influenced by Darwinism, which saw man as an organism driven by needs that he tries to satisfy under specific environmental conditions. Therefore Freud defined *"Triebe"* (drives) at the border between the somatic and the psychic. He understood psychological qualities, the developmental stages of sexuality and the ego functions as the product of a long evolutionary history in which man continuously adapted to inner and outer realities (cf. also Jones et al., 1960; Gay, 1988; Zaretzki, 2004, p. 473 ff; Whitebook, 2010, 2017).

One of the great achievements of Freud discovering psychoanalysis is undisputedly that he kept up with the natural sciences of his time, whilst also integrating so-called humanities and cultural sciences. Freud, as a young man was very interested in philosophy and other humanities before he turned to the natural sciences with a remarkably violent emotional reaction. In the laboratory at the Physiological Institute of Ernst Brücke, he got to know a strictly positivistic understanding of science that attracted him throughout his life. Nevertheless, Freud later turned away from the neurology of his time, because he recognized the limits of the methods available in the neurosciences of his time for researching the psyche. With the *Interpretation of Dreams* (1900), the birth document of psychoanalysis, he defined it as *pure psychology*. However, he continued to see himself as a physician who observed complex clinical phenomena like a natural scientist. According to Joel Whitebook (2010), his desire for a precise "empirical" examination of hypotheses and theories protected Freud from his own inclination to wild speculation. As a "philosophical physician" he was thus able to establish a new "specific science of the unconscious" - psychoanalysis.

Makari (2008) as well as Zaretzki (2004) remarkably describe how, even in the early days of psychoanalysis, Freud and his followers tried to find a way between, on the one hand, an open, innovative discussion, with constant questioning of so-called "truths" - as they characterized a scientific discourse - and, on the other hand, the search for a common identity, the specific characteristics of "psychoanalysis".

According to Makari (2008), this understanding of psychoanalysis has been a key to its success. In retrospect, it was a momentous decision of Freud's to stick to his understanding of psychoanalysis in this area of content-related and institutional tension and to resist the danger of integrating psychoanalysis either into the world of medicine or into that of "pure cultural sciences and humanities". Psychoanalysis therefore retained its autonomy as a scientific discipline. Even in 1909 Freud considered integrating psychoanalysis into the medical organization "*Internationaler Verein für medizinische Psychologie und Psychotherapie*" of August Forel or even into the "*Orden für Ethik und Kultur*". Fortunately, he decided during the Sylvester night 1910 to found his own organization, the International Psychoanalyical Association (IPA, see Falzeder, 2010). With this decision, the independence of psychoanalysis as a scientific discipline with its own research methodology and institution was protected. Afterwards, Freud always emphasized that psychoanalysis did not deserve to be "swallowed up" by medicine. Instead he said, "as a 'deep-psychology', a theory of the mental unconscious, it can become indispensable to all the sciences which are concerned with the evolution of human civilization and its major institutions such as art, religion and the social order" (Freud, 1926, p. 248).

Since the 1990s, many psychoanalysts have repeatedly raised the question of whether the developments and achievements in psychoanalysis itself, and also in neighboring sciences such as the neurosciences, are now opening new creative alternatives to cope with tendencies of retreating into the ivory tower of psychoanalytic societies on the one hand and the danger of over-adapting to an understanding of science that does not do justice to psychoanalysis as a science of the unconscious on the other. Mark Solms and the so-called neuropsychoanalysis, psychoanalytical colleagues, such as Johannes Lethonen from Finland, Mauro Manica from Italy, the research group of Wolfgang Leuschner, Stephan Hau and Tamara Fischmann at the Freud Institute in Frankfurt, have been pioneers in this field in Europe. In this volume Mark Solms and Tamara Fischmann et al. are illustrating this bridge building (Chapter 14, 15).

In another field of research, these questions are known to be particularly acute and hot: it is the so-called *outcome research in psychoanalysis*. The question of whether and how psychoanalysis should get involved in comparative studies remains controversial within the psychoanalytic community. It is especially the psychoanalytic researchers in faculties of medicine and psychology who maintain that psychoanalysis will be marginalized if it avoids comparing its effectiveness with that of other treatments, whereas psychoanalysts, especially French-speaking ones, insist that the methods derived from evidence-based medicine do not correspond to psychoanalysis as a scientific knowledge of the unconscious.

The complex epistemiological problems of empirical research in psycho-analysis remain a challenge for us all. I myself dedicated my first congress in my directorship at the Sigmund-Freud-Institut, 2002 to them. The contributions (including a controversy between André Green and Peter Fonagy) were published in the book *Plurality or Unity?* (Leuzinger-Bohleber, Dreher & Canestri., 2003).The introductory part of the *Open-Door Review* (Leuzinger-Bohleber, Arnold & Kächele, 2015) is also dedicated to this topic: Dominique Scarphone, Ricardo Bernardi, Peter Fonagy and I outline different epistemiological positions on current research in psychoanalysis.

Let me just add here a few remarks: as Feyerabend & Vetter (1976) already provocatively discussed many decades ago, at the ETH in Zurich, one objective science does not exist, it is always determined by the knowledge interests of the researchers and their social supporters (up to their financiers). He vehemently opposed "the methods compulsion" in research (Wider den Methodenzwang) in social research as well as in comparative psychotherapy research, as we intensively discussed during the so-called student revolution in the 1970s during my time as assistant at the Department of Clinical Psychology chaired by Ulrich Moser in Zürich. Today, the discourses are conducted in a different language than in the 1960s and 1970s – but the struggle for an adequate understanding of research in psychoanalysis continues and has led to exciting and challenging debates on this subject in international psychoanalysis (see also e.g. Habermas, 1971). I would like to point out just one which is taking place in Switzerland at the moment. One of the institutional successors of Feyerabend at the ETH Zurich, Michael Hampe, is reflecting with his team on the epistemiological status of psychoanalysis in an innovative way. He sees empirical outcome studies in a special area of tension, for example, between the psychoanalytic culture of treatments in private practices, which for him as a philosopher of science are connected with a *contemplative search for the truth of human life*, which should help people to reflect on the unconscious, often irrational meaning of their psychological symptoms, fantasies and conflicts in a protected, safe space within the therapeutic relationship. On the other hand, there is massive social and economic pressure to prove the effectiveness of psychoanalytic treatments, which corresponds to a *utilitarian way of thinking* that seems to dominate strongly in the world of psychotherapy in times of evidence-based medicine. In an absolutist manner, the representatives of the utilitarian zeitgeist are referring to it as "objective science" and "empirically proven truths". Hampe and his research team find such an understanding of a unified science not only problematic, but also outdated in terms of a perspective of the history of science, and describe psychoanalysis as a "science sui generis" (Guggenheim et al., 2016, p. 7).[6] Thus, from Hampe's perspective, the problem of psychoanalytic outcome research in psychoanalysis is less that it has presented too few empirical studies in order to be accepted as a "science" (*Wissenschaft*), but rather that it does not have a socially recognized position, e.g. similar to that of lawyers, who, of course, also don't refer to randomized controlled trials in their arguments while "searching for truth".

However, in this volume we will discuss time and again that such innovative epistemiological reflections on the theory of science are reminiscent of a glass bead game in the current reality of health policy: evidence-based medicine does not accept such alternative concepts of science and studies based on them. Therefore, psychoanalysis was forced to conduct randomized controlled trials. As many meta-analyses show, e.g. from the group of Falk Leichsenring, psychoanalysis has done its homework: we have enough studies in the outcomes of short-term psychodynamic therapies – but now also on long-term treatments – which show that psychoanalysis is as effective as other psychotherapies (Leichsenring et al., 2011. We have discussed the state of the art of the outcome studies in this book, based on the papers of the Sandler conference 2018 in Los Angeles, where we presented the LAC study in great detail (see Leuzinger-Bohleber et al., 2020, see also section above). Other famous outcome studies on psychoanalysis and psychoanalytic long-term therapies are the Stockholm Psychotherapy Study, the Munich Depression Study, the Helsinki Psychotherapy Study, the Tavistock Depression Study, and – from this country – the Zurich Depression Study.[7]

Psychoanalysis thus has demonstrated its outcomes in all these elaborated, costly and challenging studies although much of what is central in psychoanalysis to patients and their therapists cannot be shown in this type of outcome study (see Leuzinger-Bohleber et al., 2020). In this volume we will present such studies and their anchoring in the world of evidence-based medicine on the one hand, but also detailed case studies on the other hand which - as Michael Hampe postulates - are by no means "unscientific", but rather explore "truths" in a different way and are committed to an alternative understanding of *Wissenschaft* (science), according to a contemplative search for truth in the psychoanalytical setting. On the other hand, psychoanalysis cannot refuse the utilitarian zeitgeist, in order not to become completely marginalized in the contemporary world of medicine and mental health systems. In addition, for many of the patients who suffer extremely from their (depressive) symptoms, not only is their personal search for the idiosyncratic meaning of their lives, their self and identity essential, but also whether they can alleviate their psychological suffering and psychopathological symptoms with the help of their psychoanalytic treatments. This is especially true for chronically depressed, traumatized patients and their lives in a personal "hell".

"All these thoughts make my life hell ..." (Stromae)

Notes

1 This introduction is based on former publications, e.g. Leuzinger-Bohleber, Fischmann and Beutel, in press, and Leuzinger-Bohleber, 2021, 2021a).

2 M'Uzan, M. de (1994) "Slaves of quantity", *Psychoanalytic Quarterly*, LXXII, 2003, pp. 711–725.

3 In the LAC study we already assumed that we wanted to investigate – in the sense of a naturalistic study – long-term psychoanalytic treatments, as they are really carried out in private offices in Germany, financed by health insurance companies. Therefore, we assumed a thorough psychoanalytic training of the therapists and

required at least three years of experience after completion of their training. The additional training in David Taylor's manual then built on this "foundation of psychoanalytic knowledge" and sensitized the study therapists to specific challenges in the treatment technique of this difficult-to-treat group of patients.

It is well known that for the acceptance of outcome studies in times of evidence-based medicine it is necessary to use treatment manuals. This also applies to psychoanalytic long-term treatments. However, as we have discussed in various papers, these manuals have a different character from manuals for short-term psychoanalytic therapies. The group of chronically depressed patients especially requires a lot of creativity, originality and flexibility from the psychoanalyst to reach the patient emotionally, to initiate a therapeutic process at all as well as to work through the idiosyncratic unconscious conflicts and fantasies of the chronically depressed in the transference relationship. Nevertheless the creative psychoanalyst will need to follow specific psychoanalytic treatment techniques that are described in a "manual". The basic treatment principles are elaborated in such manuals (in the MODE Study we speak of a "Workbook") – not in the sense of a "cookbook" – but of binding basic principles based on a specific psychoanalytic understanding of the psychodynamics of depression. These basic principles are illustrated with concrete anchor examples from psychoanalyses or long-term psychoanalytic therapies.

4   David Taylor (2010) focuses in his manual mainly on the Kleinian tradition for understanding and treating severely depressed patients.
5   We cannot discuss different conceptualizations of trauma in different psychoanalytical cultures, e.g. in the French compared with the German culture but have to focus on our own understanding of trauma here (see e.g. Bohleber & Leuzinger-Bohleber, 2016).
6   For Hampe and his team it proves to be fruitful to compare, for example, the specific questions of the "truth" of psychoanalytic interpretations, as well as the outcomes of psychoanalytic treatments, with analogous strategies of the "finding of truth" of lawyers. In a recent email Hampe wrote to me: "The idea of relating psychoanalysis to jurisprudence ties in with John Forrester. In 1996 he wrote the article: 'If p, then what? Thinking in cases' in *History of the Human Sciences*" (pp. 1–25), where he referred to psychoanalysis. The Anglo-American legal system, unlike Roman law, is one that operates with precedents and does not start from the legal text first. This means that a potential crime is analogized with a precedent: Is the potential killing of P comparable to the 1965 murder of M? is the question that is asked first. Then analogies and disanalogies between the precedent and the given case are sought. Giambattista Vico, the great player of Descartes, lawyer and philosopher, wrote in his *Principles of a New Science* that finding justice in a trial is about finding out how an individual case deviates from the general descriptions of the law (Vico 1979 (Org. 1725), p. 65). In the small booklet *In the Medium of the Unconscious*, Daniel Strassberg, who wrote his doctoral thesis on Vico, and I have now combined Forrester and Vico (Guggenheim et al. 2016, p. 28f.) and interpreted psychoanalysis as follows: It thinks like the English case law in cases. First of all, there is the story of Oedipus as the 'original precedent case'. Then, in the course of the history of therapy, more and more case histories accumulate: Anna O, the Rat Man, etc. New cases are then analogized to these precedents. It is not a matter of subsumption of the new cases under the descriptions of the old ones, but of recognizing (in the sense of Vico) how the given case deviates from the precedents to which it is most similar. Thinking in cases is thus a form of recognizing the individual, the specificity of a mental illness in a narrative by learning to see it as a deviation from the known. This perhaps distinguishes psychoanalytic case histories from the others in medicine, where similarities rather than deviations are sought, although the narrative of the medical history is of course also important in somatic medicine" (Michael Hampe in an email to M. Leuzinger-Bohleber, 25.4.2020).

7 David Taylor summarizes some of the main controversial discussions of such studies, particularly those who try to fulfill the criteria of evidence-based medicine and thus use treatment manuals (2015): "On the psychoanalytic 'side' the central objection is that when the methods of empirical science (and therefore those of evidence-based medicine) are applied, something of the openness to human nature that is essential to psychoanalysis is closed down; what results is both a limited view of the human psyche and flawed therapy outcome findings" (p. 846).

References

Abbass, A., Kisely, S., & Kroenke, K. (2009). Short-term psychodynamic psychotherapy for somatic disorders: Systematic review and meta-analysis of clinical trials. *Psychotherapy and Psychosomatics*, 78, 265–274.

Blatt, S. J. (2004). *Experiences of depression: Theoretical, clinical, and research perspectives.* Washington, DC: American Psychological Association.

Blatt, S. J., & Zuroff, D. C. (2005). Empirical evaluation of the assumptions in identifying evidence based treatments in mental health. *Clinical Psychology Review*, 25(4), 459–486.

Bleichmar, H. B. (1996). Some subtypes of depression and their implications for psychoanalytic treatment. *International Journal of Psycho-Analysis*, 77, 935–961.

Bleichmar, H. (2010). Rethinking pathological mourning: Multiple types and therapeutic approaches. *The Psychoanalytic Quarterly*, 79, 71–94.

Blomberg J. (2001). Long-term outcome of long-term psychoanalytically oriented therapies: First findings of the Stockholm outcome of psychotherapy and psychoanalysis study. *Psychotherapy Research*, 11(4), 361–382.

Bodenstab, J. (2015). *Dramen der Verlorenheit: Mutter-tochter-Beziehungen in der Shoah: Zur Rezeption und zur narrativen Gestalt traumatischer erfahrungen in videozeugnissen* (Vol. 19). Göttingen: Vandenhoeck & Ruprecht.

Bohleber, W. (2005). Editorial zu der Special Issue oft he Journal Psyche "Depression. Psychoanalytische Erkundungen einer Zeitkrankheit". Zur Psychoanalyse der Depression. Erscheinungsformen-Behandlung-Erklärungsansätze. *Psyche Z Psychoanal*, 59, 781–788.

Bohleber, W. (2010). *Destructiveness, intersubjectivity, and trauma: The identity crisis of modern psychoanalysis.* London: Karnac.

Bohleber, W. (2012). *Was Psychoanalyse heute leistet. Identität und Intersubjektivität, Trauma und Therapie, Gewalt und Gesellschaft.* Stuttgart: Klett-Cotta.

Bohleber W., & Leuzinger-Bohleber, M. (2016). The special problem of interpretation in the treatment of traumatized patients. *Psychoanalytic Inquiry*, 36(1), 60–76.

Caligor, E., Kernberg, O, Clarkin, J., & Yeomans, F. E. (2018). *Psychodynamic therapy for personality pathology, treating self and interpersonal functioning.* Washington, DC: American Psychiatric Association.

Cooper, A. (1986). Toward a limited definition of psychic trauma. In: A. Rothstein (Ed.), *The reconstruction of trauma: Its significance in clinical work* (pp. 41–56). Madison, CT: International Universities Press.

Corveleyn, J., Luyten, P., Blatt, S.J., Lens-Gielis, H. (Eds.) (2013). *The theory and treatment of depression: Towards a dynamic interactionism model* (Vol. 5). London: Routledge.

Cuipers, P., Huibers, M., & Furukawa, T. (2017). The need for research on treatments of chronic depression. *JAMA Psychiatry*, 74, 242–243.

Damasio, A. R. (1994), *Descartes errors: Emotion, reason, and the human brain*. New York, NY: Penguin Group.

De Maat, S., de Jonghe, F., de Kraker, R., Leichsenring, F., Abbass, A., Luyten, P., ... & Dekker, J. (2013). The current state of the empirical evidence for psychoanalysis: A meta-analytic approach. *Harvard Review of Psychiatry*, 21, 107–137.

Driessen, E., Cuijpers, P., de Maat, S., Abbass, A., de Jonghe, F., & Dekker, J. (2010). The efficacy of short-term psychodynamic psychotherapy for depression: A meta-analysis. *Clinical Psychology Review*, 30(1), 25–36.

Edelman, G. (1987). *Neural Darwinism: The theory of neuronal group selection*. New York, NY: Basic Books.

Edelman, G. M. (1989). *The remembered present: A biological theory of consciousness*. New York, NY: Basic Books.

Ehrenberg, A. (2016). *The weariness of the self: Diagnosing the history of depression in the contemporary age*. Montreal, QC: McGill-Queen's Press.

Emde, R. N., & Leuzinger-Bohleber, M. (Eds.) (2014). *Early parenting and prevention of disorder: Psychoanalytic research at interdisciplinary frontiers*. London: Karnac.

Erikson, E. H. (1958/1993). *Childhood and society*. New York: WW Norton (German translation: Erikson, E. (1971). *Kindheit und Gesellschaft*. Stuttgart: Klett Cotta).

Falzeder, E. (2010). *Die Gründungsgeschichte der IPV und der Berliner Ortsgruppe*, lecture at the conference of the DPG and DPV: 100 Jahre Internationale Psychoanalytische Vereinigung (IPV) – 100 Jahre institutionalisierte Psychoanalyse in Deutschland, Berlin, 6 March 2010.

Fonagy, P. (2015). The effectiveness of psychodynamic psychotherapies: An update. *World Psychiatry*, 14, 137–150.

Fonagy, P., & Luyten, P. (2009). A developmental, mentalization-based approach to the understanding and treatment of borderline personality disorder. *Development and Psychopathology*, 21(4), 1355–1381.

Fonagy, P., Rost, F., Carlyle, J., McPherson, S., Thomas, R., Pasco Fearon, R. *et al.* (2015). Pragmatic randomized controlled trial of long-term psychoanalytic psychotherapy for treatment-resistant depression: The Tavistock Adult Depression Study (TADS). *World Psychiatry*, 14(3), 312–321.

Fonagy, P., Luyten P., & Allison E. (2015). Epistemic petrification and the restoration of epistemic trust: A new conceptualization of borderline personality disorder and its psychosocial treatment. *Journal of Personality Disorders*, 29(5), 575–609.

Freud, S. (1895). The neuro-psychoses of defense, *S.E.* 3.

Freud, S. (1900). The interpretation of dream, *S.E.* 2.

Freud, S. (1917). Mourning and melancholia, *S.E.* 14.

Freud, S. (1923). The ego and the id. *S.E.* 19.

Freud, S. (1926). The question of lay analysis, *S.E.* 20.

Gaensbauer, T. J. (2011). Embodied simulation, mirror neurons, and the reenactment of trauma in early childhood. *Neuropsychoanalysis*, 13, 91–107.

Feyerabend, P., & Vetter, H. (1976). *Wider den Methodenzwang: Skizze einer anarchistischen Erkenntnistheorie* (p. 107). Frankfurt: Suhrkamp.

Gallese, V. (2009). Mirror neurons, embodied simulation, and the neural basis of social identification. *Psychoanalic Dialogues*, 19, 519–536.

Gallese, V. (2013). Mirror neurons, embodied simulation and a second-person approach to mind-reading. *Cortex* 49, 2954–2956.

Grande, T., Dilg, R., Jakobsen, T., Keller, W., Krawietz, B., Langer, M. *et al.* (2009). Structural change as a predictor of long-term follow-up outcome. *Psychotherapy Research*, 19(3), 344–357.

Green, A. (2007). Pulsions de destruction et maladies somatiques. *Revue française de psychosomatique*, 2, 45–70.

Habermas, J. (1971). *Erkenntnis und Interesse* (Vol. 422). Boston, MA: Beacon Press.

Gay, P., & Berisch, K. (1988). *"Ein gottloser Jude": Sigmund Freuds Atheismus und die Entwicklung der Psychoanalyse*. Frankfurt: S. Fischer.

Guggenheim, J. Z., Hampe, M., Schneider, P., & Strassberg, D. (2016). *Im Medium des Unbewussten: Zur Theorie der Psychoanalyse*. Stuttgart: Kohlhammer Verlag.

Hagmann, G. (1995). Mourning: A review and reconsideration. *International Journal of Psychoanalysis*, 76, 909–925.

Hauser, S. T. (2008). The interplay of genes, environments, and psychoanalysis. *Journal of the American Psychoanalytic Association*, 56, 509–514.

Hill, J. (2009). Developmental perspectives on adult depression. *Psychoanalytic Psychotherapy*, 23, 200–212.

Huber, D., & Klug, G. (2016). Münchner Psychotherapiestudie. *Psychotherapeut*, 61 (6), 462–467.

Huhn, M., Tardy, M., Spineli, L. M., Kistling, W., Förstl, L. H., Pitschel-Walsh, G. *et al.* (2014). Efficacy of pharmacotherapy and psychotherapy for adult psychiatric disorders: A systematic overview of meta-analyses. *JAMA Psychiatry*, 71, 706–715.

Jiménez, J. P. (2019). *The role of early trauma in depression*. Unpublished paper given at the Joseph Sandler Conference in Buenos Aires, May 2019.

Jiménez, J. P., Botto, A., & Fonagy, P. (2021). *Etiopathogenic theories and models in depression*. Cham, Switzerland: Springer.

Jones, E., Jones, K., & Meili-Dworetzki, G. (1960). *Das Leben und Werk von Sigmund Freud* (Vol. 3). Bern: Huber.

Kächele, H., & Thomä, H. (2000). *Lehrbuch der psychoanalytischen Therapie Band 3 Forschung/Psychoanalytic Practice Vol 3 Research*. Ulm: Ulmer Textbank (new edition in preparation).

Kächele, H., Leuzinger-Bohleber, M., Buchheim, A., & Thomä, H. (2006). Amalie X. – ein deutscher Musterfall. In: H. Thomä & H. Kächele (Eds.), *Psychoanalytische Therapie. Forschung* (pp. 121–174). Berlin: Springer.

Keilson, H. (1991). Sequentielle Traumatisierung bei Kindern. Ergebnisse einer Follow-up-Untersuchung. In: *Schicksale der Verfolgten* (pp. 98–109). Berlin, Heidelberg: Springer.

Khan, M. (1964). Ego distortion, cumulative trauma, and the role of reconstruction in the analytic situation. *International Journal of Psycho-Analysis*, 45, 272–279.

Knekt, P., Lindfors, O., Laaksonen, M. A., Renlund, C., Haaramo, P., Härkänen, T., Helsinki Psychotherapy Study Group. (2011). Quasi-experimental study on the effectiveness of psychoanalysis, long-term and short-term psychotherapy on psychiatric symptoms, work ability and functional capacity during a 5-year follow-up. *Journal of Affective Disorders*, 13, 37–47.

Knox, J. (2009). Mirror neurons and embodied simulation in the development of archetypes and self-agency. *Journal of Analytical Psychology*, 54, 307–323.

Krystal, H. (1968/2015). *Integration and self-healing: Affect, trauma, alexithymia*. London: Routledge

Lakoff, G., & Johnson, M. (1999). *Philosophy in the flesh: The embodied mind and its challenge to western thought*. New York, NY: Basic Books.

Lane, R., Ryan, L., Nadel, L., & Greenberg, L. (2015). Memory reconsolidation, emotional arousal, and the process of change in psychotherapy: New insights from brain science. *Behavioral and Brain Sciences*, 38, 1–64.

Laub, D. (2005). From speechlessness to narrative: The cases of Holocaust historians and of psychiatrically hospitalized survivors. *Literature and Medicine*, 24(2), 253–265.

Leichsenring, F. (2008). Effectiveness of long-term psychodynamic psychotherapy. *JAMA*. 300(13), 1551–1565.

Leichsenring, F., & Rabung, S. (2011). Long-term psychodynamic psychotherapy in complex mental disorders: Update of a meta-analysis. *British Journal of Psychiatry*, 199, 15–22.

Leuzinger-Bohleber, M. (2008). Biographical truths and their clinical consequences: Understanding "embodied memories" in a third psychoanalysis with a traumatized patient recovered from serve poliomyelitis. *International Journal of Psychoanalysis*, 89, 1165–1187.

Leuzinger-Bohleber, M. (2012).Changes in dreams: From a psychoanalysis with a traumatised, chronic depressed patient. In: P. Fonagy, H. Kächele, M. Leuzinger-Bohleber & D. Taylor (Eds.), *The significance of dreams: Bridging clinical and extraclinical research in psychoanalysis* (pp. 49–85). London: Karnac Books.

Leuzinger-Bohleber, M. (2015). *Finding the body in the mind: Embodied memories, trauma, and depression.* London: Karnac.

Leuzinger-Bohleber, M. (2015a). Working with severely traumatized, chronically depressed analysands. *International Journal of Psychoanalysis*, 96, 611–636.

Leuzinger-Bohleber, M.(2021). Contemporary psychodynamic theories on depression. In: J. P. Jiménez, A. Botto, & P. Fonagy (Eds.), *Etiopathogenic theories and models in depression* (pp. 78–104). Cham, Switzerland: Springer.

Leuzinger-Bohleber, M. (2021a). Psychoanalyse als plurale Wissenschaft des Unbewußten. Allgemeine Zeitschrift für Philosophie. *Heft*, 46(2), 253–267.

Leuzinger-Bohleber, M., & Pfeifer, R. (2002). Remembering a depressive primary object? Memory in the dialogue between psychoanalysis and cognitive science. *International Journal of Psychoanalysis*, 83, 3–33.

Leuzinger-Bohleber, M., Stuhr, U., Rüger, B., & Beutel, M. (2003). How to study the "quality of psychoanalytic treatments" and their long-term effects on patients' well-being: A representative, multi-perspective follow-up study. *International Journal of Psychoanalysis*, 84(2), 263–290.

Leuzinger-Bohleber, M., Dreher, A. U., & Canestri, J. (Eds.) (2003). *Pluralism and unity? Methods of research in psychoanalysis.* London: International Psychoanalytical Association (The International Psychoanalysis Library).

Leuzinger-Bohleber, M., Arnold, S., & Kächele, H. (Eds) (2015/2019). *An open-door review of outcome and process studies in psychoanalysis.* London: International Psychoanalytical Association.

Leuzinger-Bohleber, M., Kallenbach, L., Assenburg, L., Lebiger-Vogel, J., & Rickmeyer, C. (2017). Psychoanalytische Fokaltheraien für Patienten mit Zwangsstörungen? *Psyche-Z Psychoanal*, 71(98), 704–732.

Leuzinger-Bohleber, M., Hautzinger, M., Fiedler, G., Keller, W., Bahrke, U., Kallenbach, L., … & Küchenhoff, H. (2019). Outcome of psychoanalytic and cognitive-behavioural long-term therapy with chronically depressed patients: A controlled trial with preferential and randomized allocation. *The Canadian Journal of Psychiatry*, 64(1), 47–58.

Leuzinger-Bohleber, M., Kaufhold, J., Kallenbach, L., Ernst, M., Keller, W., ... & Beutel, M. (2019a). How to measure sustained psychic transformations in long-term treatments of chronically depressed patients: Symptomatic and structural changes in the LAC Depression Study of the outcome of cognitive-behavioural and psychoanalytic long-term treatments. *International Journal of Psychoanalysis*, 100(1), 99–127.

Leuzinger-Bohleber, M., Solms, M., & Arnold, S. E. (Eds.) (2020). *Outcome research and the future of psychoanalysis: Clinicans and researchers in dialogue*. London: Routledge.

Leuzinger-Bohleber, M., Fischmann, T., & Beutel, M. (in press). *Analytischen Langzeitpsychotherapien von chronisch depressiven Patienten (LAC Manual)*. Göttingen: Hogrefe Verlag.

Levine, H. B., Reed, G. S., & Scarfone, D. (2013). *Unrepresented states and the construction of meaning: Clinical and theoretical contributions*. London:Karnac.

Liliengren, P. (2019). Available: www.research-gate.net/pulication/317335876. (Comprehensive compilation of randomized controlled trials (RCTs) involving psychodynamic treatment and interventions.)

Loch, W. (1967). Psychoanalytische Aspekte zur Pathogenese und Struktur depressivpsychotischer Zustandsbilder. *Psyche-Z Psychoanal*, 21, 758–779

Makari, G. (2008). *Revolution in mind: The creation of psychoanalysis*. Melbourne: Melbourne University Publishing.

Marshall, K. (2009). The embodied self: Thinking psychoanalytically in a time of "science". *Journal of Analytical Psychology*, 54, 677–696.

Mentzos, S. (1995). *Depression und Manie. Psychodynamik und Therapie affektiver Störungen*. Göttingen: Vandenhoeck & Ruprecht.

Minkmar, N. (2022). Ins Licht. *Süddeutsche Zeitung*, 13 January, p. 9.

Moser, U., & Zeppelin, I. (1996). *Der geträumte Traum*. Stuttgart: Kohlhammer.

Moussavi, S., Chatterji, S., Verdes, E., Tandon, A., Patel, V., Ustun, B. (2007). Depression, chronic diseases, and decrements in health: Results from the World Health Surveys. *The Lancet*, 370, 851–858.

Nadel, L., & Moscovitch, M. (1997). Memory consolidation, retrograde amnesia and the hippocampal complex. *Current opinion in neurobiology*, 7(2), 217–227.

Negele, A., Kaufhold, J., Kallenbach, L., & Leuzinger-Bohleber, M. (2015). Childhood trauma and its relation to chronic depression in adulthood. *Depression Research and Treatment*, 2015, 2–11.

Peterson, B., Leuzinger-Bohleber, M., Fischmann, T., Ambresin, G., Axmacher, N., Lerner, R. *et al.* (2019). Multi-level outcome study of psychoanalyses of chronically depressed patients with early trauma (MODE): Initial Phase. Unpublished Research Application to the IPA /ApsaA.

Pfeifer, R., & Bongard, J. (2007). *How the body shapes the way we think: A new view of intelligence*. Cambridge, MA: The MIT Press.

Radebold, H., Heuft, G., & Fooken, I. (Eds.). (2006). *Kindheiten im Zweiten Weltkrieg: Kriegserfahrungen und deren Folgen aus psychohistorischer Perspektive*. Weinheim: Beltz Juventa.

Ryan, L., Hoscheidt, S., & Nadel, L. (2008). Perspectives on episodic and semantic memory retrieval. In: E. Dere, A. Easton, J. Huston & L. Nadel (Eds.), *Handbook of episodic memory (Handbook of behavioral neuroscience)* (pp. 5–18). Amsterdam: Elsevier.

Reed, G. (2013). An empty mirror: reflections on nonrepresentation. In: H. B. Levine, G. S. Reed & D. Scarfone (Eds.), *Unrepresented states and the construction of meaning: Clinical and theoretical contributions* (pp. 18–41). London: Karnac.

Sandell, R., Blomberg, J., Lazar, A., Carlsson, J., Broberg, J., & Schubert, J. (2001). Unterschiedliche Langzeitergebnisse von Psychoanalysen und Langzeitpsychotherapien. Aus der Forschung des Stockholmer Psychoanalyse-und Psychotherapieprojekts. *Psyche*, 55(3), 277–310.

Scarfone, D. (2013). A brief introduction to the work of Jean Laplanche. *International Journal of Psychoanalysis*, 94, 545–566.

Shapiro, S. A. (2009). A rush to action: Embodiment, the analyst's subjectivity, and the interpersonal experience. *Studies in Gender and Sexuality*, 10, 93–103.

Shedler, J. (2010). The efficacy of psychodynamic psychotherapy. *American Psychologist*, 65, 98–109.

Shedler, J. (2015). Where is the evidence for "evidence-based" therapy? *The Journal of Psychological Therapies in Primary Care*, 4, 47–59.

Squire, L. R., & Alvarez, P. (1995). Retrograde amnesia and memory consolidation: A neurobiological perspective. *Current opinion in neurobiology*, 5(2), 169–177.

Steinert, C., Hofmann, M., Kruse, J., Leichsenring, F. (2014). Relapse rates after psychotherapy for depression: Stable long-term effects? A meta-analysis. *Journal of Affective Disorders*, 168, 107–118.

Taylor, D. (2010). Tavistock-Manual der Psychoanalytischen Psychotherapie. *Psyche-Z Psychoanal*, 64, 833–886.

Trivedi, R. B., Nieuwsma J. A., & Williams J. W. (2011). Examination of the utility of psychotherapy for patients with treatment resistant depression: A systematic review. *Journal of General Internal Medicine*, 26, 643–650.

Vivona, J. M. (2009). Embodied language in neuroscience and psychoanalysis. *Journal of the American Psychoanalytic Association*, 57, 1327–1360.

Whitebook, J. (2010). *Sigmund Freud: A philosophical physician*, Vortrag an der 11. Joseph Sandler Research Conference: Persisting Shadows of Early and Later Trauma, Frankfurt,7 February 2010.

Whitebook, J. (2017). *Freud: an Intellectual Biography*. New York: Cambridge University Press.

Will, H. (1994). Zur Phänomenologie der Depression aus psychoanalytischer Sicht. *Psyche-Z Psychoanal*, 48, 361–385.

Zaretzki, E. (2021). *The big lie*. London: London Review of Books.

2 From acedia to melancholy

Sadness in the presence of God

J. N. Despland

Introduction

The word "depression" is recent in psychiatry: it dates from the end of the 19th century in Germany, the beginning of the 20th century in the USA via a Swiss psychiatrist, Adolphe Meyer at John Hopkins, and even later in France. The depression "epidemic" that we know is even more modern. It dates back to the 1970s, during the development of antidepressants, with a second wave, unfortunately a fashionable term, since the 1980s and linked to the development of SSRIs.

The word "melancholy" has a richer and more complex history: it is the subject of medical, psychological, philosophical, literary and art historical discussions. This text deals with a particular aspect of this history associated since the 4th century with what is called acedia. Acedia, which can be defined as a spiritual illness, is associated with the life of a man, Evagrius the Pontic, who lived from 345 to 399 and ended his life as a hermit in the desert next to the Nile delta, where Christian monasticism was to develop (Guillaumont, 2004).

Evagrius is at the origin of a fascinating body of texts, translated into French by Antoine Guillaumont (Evagrius the Pontic, 1971, 1998). He describes a doctrine, defining both the framework of life and the rules that apply to a hermit in search of God. At the same time, he constructs a true psychopathology of the life experience that results from this framework and the application of these rules. This psychopathology is dedicated to the demons, also called evil thoughts. There are eight of them, including acedia. This one will have an eventful destiny. It will be confused with sadness and laziness for theological reasons, and will then have a complex relationship with melancholy, both on their dark and their light side.

Evagrius

Evagrius was born in 345 in Ibora in Pontus, in the north of present-day Turkey. As the son of a bishop in a rural community, he was destined for an ecclesiastical career. In 380 he left his homeland to go to Constantinople. He

DOI: 10.4324/9781003279297-2

studied and seems to have been very successful as a rhetorician in his preaching against heresy. Enjoying this social success, he led a relatively worldly life.

It was then, according to the historian Palladius, that a break occurred in his life following a love affair: he fell in love with the wife of a high official, the prefect of the city, who responded to his passion. Fearing for his soul, and perhaps also for his life, Evagrius is drawn into this situation by a dream in which an angel, disguised as a friend, advises him to leave. He leaves Constantinople for Jerusalem. There he is welcomed by Melania of Rome and Ruffin, both having adopted the ascetic life and founded convents.

During his stay, he fell ill, but the doctors were unable to diagnose and cure him. He then confessed to Melanie what seemed to be agitating his thoughts, namely the love affair with Constantinople and the conflict with his religious aspirations. She encourages him to respect his vocation, while his symptoms fade. He then abandoned Jerusalem for Nitria in 383, where he resided for two years, and then withdrew to the Kellia desert (Bridel 1988, Guillaumont 1965, 1988), located 70 kilometres south of Alexandria, to join other monks and admirers of Origen. He led the life of a semi-anchorite, dividing his time between manual work and prayer. He worked as a copyist, but also wrote many texts. He died in 399, aged 54.

The doctrine: *hesychia, hypomonè, praktike* and *apatheia*

His doctrine of *hesychia* (life in solitude and inner peace) witnesses to the monastic environment in which he lived (Evagrius the Pontic 1971, 1998). *Hesychia* refers to the state of perfect tranquillity in which the monk must find himself in order to attain *apatheia*, impassibility and access to beatitude, seeing God. But this aspiration is not simple and requires the anchorite to rid himself of any representation associated with desire. He thus lives in *anachoresis*. He must remain celibate, or better still, continent. He must live in poverty. To combat the temptation to leave his cell and to maintain the virtue of "perseverance", *hypomonè*, the monk must apply himself unceasingly to manual work.

More concretely, the life of the anchorite is marked by an apparently very repetitive activity. He must remain in his cell and provide for his needs through his work, essentially basketry. Prayer occupies the rest of his time. The term "prayer" covers a variety of activities, including regular services and the recitation of formulas from Scripture. Every Saturday evening a service is held for anchorites from the same hermitage or from neighbouring hermitages, the synapse.

From *hysechia* to *apatheia*, the path is arduous. The outer calm of *hysechia* does not immediately bring inner calm, which is difficult to achieve. Between the two lies what Evagrius calls *praktike*, "the spiritual method that purifies the passionate part of the soul". Indeed, the monk who has withdrawn to the desert no longer has to fight against men and their agitation, but he has to confront otherwise formidable adversaries, the demons. Very importantly, the demons' weapons are the monk's evil thoughts, *logismoi*, which they do not provoke, but which they use.

How can demons provoke these thoughts in the desert, where the objects that usually serve as their intermediaries are lacking? They act by using "representations of sensible objects". And the reactivation of the representation, i.e. the image, is enough to bring up memories, which are themselves associated with other images. Evagrius thus makes it clear that the solitude of the anchorite, characterised by the absence of tempting objects, does not suppress desire. On the contrary, desire is all the more intense and vivid when the object is absent. The monk discovers that he is inhabited by thoughts, desires and feelings that the demons use and that hinder his encounter with God.

Acedia

Bad thoughts burst into the monk's mind and disturb his peace of mind by offering him images, representations, stimulating his imagination, recalling certain memories. The adversaries to be fought are therefore these inner thoughts that come to disturb the soul. Described in very suggestive ways by Evagrius, there are eight bad thoughts (Evagre, Traité pratique 6):

> Eight are in all the generic thoughts which include all thoughts: the first is that of gluttony, then comes that of fornication, the third is that of avarice, the fourth that of sadness, the fifth that of anger, the sixth that of acedia, the seventh that of vainglory, the eighth that of pride.

Of the eight evil thoughts, *acedia* is the most original and interesting. The word acedia comes from the classical Greek *akêdia*, which means "negligence", "indifference", or "sorrow". Rarely mentioned in secular Greek writings, sometimes in the Bible, *acedia* is mentioned by Athanasius of Alexandria in his *Life of Antony*, as well as by Origen, but in a much less specific way.

The acedious person experiences an interminable, stagnant time, with no opening to the future. The narrowness of his cell also sends him back to a heavy solitude. For these two reasons, it is difficult for him to stay still and the agitation is difficult to contain. The expectation then turns into disgust for the place where he is, the life he leads, the work he does; for the brothers too: nobody loves him, nobody comes to console him. And the bad memories are awakened. Dislike becomes bitterness. The monk then has only one desire, that of fleeing, of deserting what puts him in this state. The acedious person can also be invaded by an unpleasant torpor, against which he struggles unsuccessfully and which leads to an agitated sleep. In short, feelings of heaviness, interminable time, boredom and motor restlessness, disgust, inconsolable sadness, desire to escape and torpor are the cardinal symptoms of acedia. We will discuss the links between acedia and melancholy in more detail.

In the texts of Evagrius the Pontic, acedia is associated with the "Midday Demon". This reference is taken from v. 6 of Psalm 90 of the Septuagint Bible. Evagrius applies the epithet *barytatos* to this 'demon of the middle of the day', the most burdensome, where the figurative sense (painful) competes with the literal sense: it strikes at the hot hours of the day, when the sun is at its zenith and becomes overwhelming.

Unlike the other vices, the demon of acedia is not associated with any specific representation, like the other bad thoughts, sadness or gluttony for example. For this reason, Evagrius also says that "the demon of noon has the habit of enveloping the whole soul and of suffocating the intellect" and that it "is not immediately followed by any other". As Hélène Prigent (2005) points out, acedia would thus designate the demonic mechanism itself, the activity of thought, the imagination itself: passion of passion, passion squared, even white passion, by allusion to the white martyrdom of monks. As such, it embodies the supreme temptation against *hysechia*.

The fate of acedia

Bad thoughts, particularly acedia, were to become extraordinarily successful: the eight *logismoi* were to become seven deadly sins and acedia was to be associated with three other notions, sadness, laziness and melancholy, to finally disappear as such (Larue 2001).

In Evagrius' texts, as in Cassian's, acedia and sadness are clearly distinguished from each other. They coexist in the list of the eight bad thoughts and their respective definitions do not allow them to be confused. Gregory the Great, pope from 590 to 604, puts pride in the foreground and transforms the eight bad thoughts into a list of seven deadly sins. Acedia disappears and is absorbed by sadness and its descendants: bitterness, despair, instability, worry and idleness. St Thomas would confirm this reading a few centuries later. For what reason? It seems that both Gregory and St Thomas wish to get rid of such an ambiguous sin, which has the formidable prestige of the spirit, which can reach perfect men, and therefore cannot be a mortal sin. Scholastic theology thus insisted on its most spiritual meaning: according to Gregory and St Thomas, whom we have just quoted, acedia appears as a sin reserved for "perfect men", anchorites, monks.

The evolution of acedia into laziness is first seen in Cassian. A travelling father, author in the 420s of *Institutions cénobitiques et Conférences* which depict and organise monastic life, he exported and inflected the teaching of the Fathers of Egypt. Probably more sensitive to the difficulties of community life than to those of *anachoresis*, acedia is transformed into laziness. Later, the Church reinforced this more popular, less spiritual version, which identified *acedia* with an inclination towards sloth. It is less opposed to the joy of contemplating God than to the zeal to serve him. Thus, from the 13th century onwards, acedia ceased to be a monastic vice and the accusation of laziness gradually spread to all social and economic life. In this movement of secularisation, it is associated with sleepiness, negligence, lack of perseverance, a form of laziness and sterile idleness that is opposed to the bourgeois values associated with work. Finally, it should be remembered that in the current Catholic catechism, it is laziness that appears in the list of the seven deadly sins.

Acedia and melancholia

If acedia in its lazy form becomes secularised, we are also witnessing a form of medicalisation of acedia when it becomes confused with melancholy. In the Middle Ages, both in religious and literary texts, we see a superimposition of acedia and melancholy. Acedia and melancholy are completely confused and are the clinical manifestation of the state of sin (Clair 2007, Hersant 2005, Jouanna 2007, Larue, 2001).

What are we to make of this? First of all, it is clear that theological and medical symptoms overlap: disgust with life, a feeling of collapse and abandonment, a mixture of torpor and agitation, and time slowing down. However, we do not find in Evagrius any allusion to the disease, to black bile and to the temperament it induces, even though he has a very extensive classical culture and knowledge of Greek authors. Moreover, theology has always made a clear distinction between sin and disease. Thus, many authors emphasise that acedia can have a pathological side distinct from the moral side. How did acedia and melancholy come to be confused?

From the 13th century onwards, confessors sought to associate the sinful conduct of sinners with recognisable physical traits. For example, in specialist manuals, "dry and earthy" Christians are mentioned as potential sinners. Priests thus come to designate vice as an object of natural science in the same way that physicians associate the mental disorder of their patients with a particular physical substratum. In this regard, an impressive description of Hildegard of Bingen (1098–1179), a German Benedictine mystic nun, canonised by Benedict XVI in 2012 and named a doctoress of the Church after Catherine of Siena, Teresa of Avila and Teresa of Lisieux (de Bingen, 1903/2005), can be quoted.

Hildegard of Bingen

> The melancholic is truly a fallen creature who bears all the traces of his blackness: born from the very breath of the snake, the melancholic, whose brain is fat, [...] have a dark complexion in their face, so that even their eyes are inflamed and viper-like, and their veins are firm and thick, containing thick black blood [...].

According to Panofsky (Klibansky, Panofsky and Saxl 1964/1989), this development could be linked to the resurgence in the Middle Ages of the theory of temperaments, which is reflected in a very great interest in the relationship between the soul and the body. For acedia it is a relationship between the spiritual and the corporeal, for melancholy between the emotional and the somatic. The difference between a disease of the body that affects the soul and a disease of the soul that affects the body becomes blurred. This condensation is also evident in the iconographic tradition of melancholy and acedia, with the classic figure with the bent head being associated with both acedia and melancholy (Prigent 2007).

Melancholy and acedia thus share their dark side, but both can take on a positive value. At the dawn of the Renaissance and with the development of humanism (Petrarch, Marcile Ficino, for example), the rediscovery of classical authors, Plato and Aristotle, brought the ancient conception of melancholy back to the forefront, in particular the famous Problem XXX by the pseudo Aristotle (Aristotle 2004), which associates melancholy and genius through a reflection on the imagination (*fantasia*).

Aristotle, Problem XXX

Why is it that all those who were outstanding in philosophy, politics, poetry or the arts were obviously melancholic, some to the point of contracting diseases caused by black bile, like Heracles in the heroic myths? ... Many other heroes seem to have been afflicted by the same condition: among those closest to us, this was the case of Empedocles, Plato, Socrates and a large number of famous people, as well as most poets.

For Marcile Ficino, philosophical speculation is only accessible if the soul has freed itself from the sensible world, i.e. from the body, making it die within itself. But in this operation of sublimation, he will come up against melancholy. Doubting himself, he confided in his friend Calvacanti who confirmed that it was to Saturn that Ficino owed his greatest qualities, memory, audacity, intelligence and wisdom. In the three books of *De vita triplici*, published in 1497, Ficino definitively consecrated *melancolia generosa* as a unique gift in which the bile raises the soul to the understanding of the highest things.

Although these ideas spread slowly in Germany, it was a philosopher interested in occultism, Aggripa of Netesheim, who spread Neo-Platonism there. He describes three forms of melancholy. *Melancholia imaginationis* governs the lower demons and allows the most uneducated men to become painters or architects. It also rules over natural disasters, comets and rainbows. *Melancholia rationis* allows philosophers, doctors and orators to gain knowledge through reason. The *melancholia mentis*, the highest, reveals the law of God. It was Durer who portrayed the two facets of melancholy in his famous engraving *Melencolia 1* in 1417, possibly dedicated to *melancholia imaginationis*, and which includes both the classical iconography of melancholy and that of geometry (Klibansky, Panofsky and Saxl 1964/1989).

If acedia is stigmatizing, in its original definition as well as in the secularised form of laziness or the dramatic form of the melancholic habitus, it nevertheless retains a very special status. It is a pure sin of the mind, it is not associated with any representation and can reach perfect men. And for this reason, it is not a mortal sin according to St Thomas. More fundamentally, it is a stage, a necessary testing of the monk, which must precede the beatitude, described as a formless light with which the intellect is clothed. Acedia thus has a redemptive value.

Classical melancholy and acedia thus have in common that they portray a divided man, in whom the imagination, evil thoughts, threaten his sense of unity. Unity between the body and the intellect for Aristotelian melancholy, unity of man in his quest for the knowledge of God for Evagrian acedia. But both are ambivalent. Both have a dark side and a light side, genius in philosophy, politics, poetry or the arts for the melancholy of Problem XXX, redemption and beatitude for acedia (Larue 2001).

Acedia today?

Finally, in the 15th and 16th centuries, when the Reformation contributed to the erasure of patristic and scholastic sources, melancholy devoured acedia. By the mid-fifteenth century, in his Anatomy of Melancholy, Robert Burton only spoke of "religious melancholy". In the 19th century, a fully medicalised description can be found in a work by Brière de Boismont devoted to suicide (1845/1956). It was the Romantic movement that gave it some lustre, notably in Baudelaire works.

Acedia still exists, for example in the lexicon of the website of the Catholic Church of France (www.eglise.catholique.fr) and gives rise to many theological comments. More debatable, many articles, including the one on Wikipedia, suggest that acedia has an existence in itself and that it is sufficient to specify its contemporary forms. This point of view assumes a quasi-teleological vision of history, whereas the encounter between acedia, laziness, sadness or melancholy is due to multiple factors. The historical context determines new meanings and new links in each period.

The "Midday Demon", mentioned in verse 6 of Psalm 90 and assimilated to acedia by Evagrius, has a nice posterity. In the first place, philologists consider that this expression results from an error in the translation of the Septuagint Bible: *shêd*: demon – instead of *yâshûd*: which devastates, an error taken up in the Vulgate. Nevertheless, we recall the success of Paul Bourget's 1914 novel, *Le démon de midi* (Bourget 1914), which gave this expression its more recent meaning, associated with a mid-life crisis, a fervent Catholic and married man giving in to temptation after having found a youthful love. Paul Bourget was also an avid reader of Freud and helped introduce him to France. A more recent text by Paul-Laurent Assoun, Le Démon de Midi (Assoun 2010), updates this concept by explicitly assimilating it to the drive and its bodily roots.

More specifically, the notion of acedia is inseparable from its conditions of emergence, historical first of all, but also from the framework associated with it (Guillaumont, 2004):

Evagrius analyses thoughts in a sort of pure state, in privileged experimental conditions, which are those of anachoresis, where they act independently of the presence of objects; his analysis is nonetheless of general value, because, in any case, it is not the objects that tempt us, but the thoughts they awaken in us.

Anne Larue (2001) gives a contemporary definition of acedia today, which questions the actuality of this notion:

> When we get up, when we smoke, when we snack, when we answer the phone instead of concentrating: acedia. When you work like a madman on your line, until you die of stress for no apparent reason: acedia. When you rush sterilely to a shop because you suddenly absolutely need a pack of envelopes or a set of paper clips, supposedly for work: acedia. When you think about sex, in the solitude of your work, when the black-printed whiteness of the paper is no longer enough to survive: acedia. When you can't stay in peace in a room, thus making not only your own misfortune, but also the misfortune of all men: acedia. It is desire that is at stake, desire as an anti-social force. It "ignores exchange [and] recognises only theft and gift", desire as a figure of Eros, a primitive energy, a winged god mythologically born even before Heaven and Earth. (147)

References

Aristotle (2004). *Problème XXX* (trans. A. Carbone et B. Fau). Paris: Allia.

Assoun, P-L. (2010). Le midi passionné. Le corps dans le démon de midi. *Champ psy*, 57, 29–41

Bourget, P. (1914). *Le démon de midi*. Paris:Plon-Nourrit.

Bridel, Ph. (1988). L'installation dans le désert. *Histoire et Archéologie*, 163, 16–19.

Brière de Boismont, A. (1956). *Du suicide et de la folie suicide considérés dans leurs rapports avec la statistique, la médecine et la philosophie*. Paris: Germaire-Baillière.

Clair, J. & Kopp, R. (Eds.) (2007). *De la mélancolie. Les entretiens de la Fondation des Treilles*. Paris: Gallimard.

de Bingen, H. (1903/2005). *Les causes et les remèdes*. Grenoble: Jérôme Millon.

Evagre le Pontique (1971). *Traité pratique ou le moine I et II* (trans. A. Guillaumont). Paris: Les Editions du Cerf.

Evagre le Pontique (1998). *Sur les pensées* (trans. A. Guillaumont). Paris: Les Editions du Cerf.

Guillaumont, A. (1965). Premières fouilles au site des kellia (Basse-Egypte). *Comptes-rendus des séances de l'Académie des Inscriptions et Belles-Lettres*, 109, 218–225.

Guillaumont, A. (1988). Les moines des Kellia au IV–V e siècle. *Histoire et Arché-ologie*, 163, 6–13.

Guillaumont, A. (2004). *Un philosophe au désert. Evagre le Pontique*. Paris: Vrin.

Hersant, Y. (2005). *Mélancolies – de l'Antiquité au XXe siècle*. Paris: Robert Laffont.

Jouanna, J. (2007). Aux racines de la mélancolie: la médecine grecque est-elle mélancolique? In: J. Clair & R. Kopp (Eds.), *De la mélancolie. Les entretiens de la Fondation des Treilles* (pp. 11–51). Paris: Gallimard.

Klibansky, R. ., Panofsky, E., & Saxl, F. (1964). *Saturne et la mélancolie*. Paris: Gallimard, 1989.

Larue, A. (2001). *L'autre mélancolie. Acedia, ou les chambres de l'esprit*. Paris: Hermann.

Prigent, H. (2005). *Mélancolie. Les métamorphoses de la dépression*. Paris: Gallimard.

Prigent, H. (2007). Mélancolie antique: une philosophie de l'image. In: J. Clair & R. Kopp (Eds.), *De la mélancolie. Les entretiens de la Fondation des Treilles* (pp. 75–93). Paris: Gallimard, 2007.

3 The unpast core of depression

Dominique Scarfone

Depression, as we know, comes in different forms, ranging from melancholia, with its delusions of shame and guilt, to essential depression, presenting a psychic desert. In between, there is a wide variety of clinical presentations that evade rigid nosographic classification. Yet, one would like to find some common denominator that is not only clinically descriptive, but also helps understand how analytical treatment operates. The notion of "dark side", which was the theme of this conference, incited me to continue my reflection on one such possible denominator: the temporal dimension, which I had begun approaching many years ago through the notion of "actual time" which I also call "the *unpast*" (Scarfone, 2006; 2015). When I started to work on the present chapter, I was in fact astonished to realize that until now, I had given little space to depression in my writings on the *unpast*, a problem which has everything to do with psychic temporality!

My present reflection was, so to speak, put in gear by a rich book, *Les bien-faits de la dépression* ("The beneficial side of depression"), by Pierre Fédida, a well-known French analyst and professor who drew creatively from his phenomenological training with Binswanger, and whom I wish to cite briefly.

Writes Fédida:

> The common experience of the depressed state could consist of a single sensation: the almost physical sensation of annihilation. This sensation is barely an affect that one experiences, and it seems very far removed from the perception of suffering experienced by the subject. It is rather similar to an immobilization, to an impediment to feel the slightest movement of internal and external life, to the abolition of all daydreaming and all desire. Thought, action and language seem to be taken over by a violence of emptiness.
>
> (Fédida, 2001, pp. 6–7)

The introductory phrases quoted above are followed by many others, all very illuminating for whoever works with depressed patients. For example:

> in the most trivial expressions of everyday humanity, the depressed state is, after all, common and familiar: it is that of the "de-human" (*déshumain*).

DOI: 10.4324/9781003279297-3

This state does not boil down to isolation from others or the withdrawal of the simplest communication. It is the human appearance itself that fades away.

(op. cit., p. 7)

Fédida immediately contrasts this state with "what is called psychic life", which makes him wonder if it is not "precisely this essential human appearance with which humanity recognizes itself every day". So that: "The depressed state would reveal in hollow this psychic life, as soon as it comes to be lacking" (p. 8).

So, if depression consists in an erasure of psychic life itself, the question soon arises of how much of it can be represented psychically. I suggest that, while acknowledging the multifactorial aspect of any depression, it is useful to suspend any idea of *additive* causality – for instance, one where traumatic or other factors come on top of a biological predisposition. I propose this suspension in order to try and think things as a whole, and revolving around *the central axis of time*.

The temporal dimension

If I were asked what I would like to add to the three metapsychological points of view proposed by Freud (topographic, dynamic and economic), it is not adaptation that would come to mind. This point of view, once proposed by Hartmann, may be useful, but I find that it is not a *metapsychological* point of view; it is rather a psychological or a sociological one. *Time*, on the other hand, would appear to me as the appropriate "fourth dimension" of metapsychology. Freud himself, in the last phase of his work, was sorry for not having given this dimension all the attention it deserved (Freud, 1933, p. 74).

I propose that, alongside the economic point of view, the temporal dimension offers Freudian metapsychology its most solid base. In my view, indeed, the economic and the temporal points of view designate the most *meta-* or, if one prefers, the least imaginary dimensions of metapsychology. For while topographical and dynamic presentations easily lend themselves to *metaphorical* images, and even operate altogether as metaphors themselves, quantity (or energy) and psychic temporality are the real thing. To be sure, as Henri Bergson (1895) was able to show more than a century ago, we constantly speak of time in spatial terms because this is the only way we can make a subjective representation of it. But one must insist that, contrary to topographic and dynamic descriptions – where agencies with opposing interests clash within a psychic "space" or "apparatus" that are purely metaphoric – temporality as such (and quantity as such) do not operate as metaphors, if only because they do not lend themselves easily to representation; yet, we could not do without them in our conception of psychic events (see Scarfone, 2015).

The axis of temporality makes it possible to describe both continuity and difference between the various clinical pictures of depression. At one end, we have melancholia with its delusional (hence representational) productions, while, at the other extreme, essential depression displays a dearth of representations (Marty, 1968). In Freud's masterful description of melancholia, we can see for instance how metaphorization is not only possible but gives us a rich and effective psychic grip, so valuable for our therapeutic endeavor. Think for instance of the shadow of the object falling on the ego, which points at a rich psychic dramaturgy. On the other hand, in non-melancholic depressions, with essential depression at their extreme, metaphors are either totally absent or they appear rather conventional and repetitive: black holes, bottomless pits, etc. This is not because clinicians lack imagination or vocabulary, but because, as Fédida points out, the depressive experience itself involves a psychic erasure, a paralysis of the metaphorical function.

Regardless of the images it evokes, the real lived experience of most forms of severe depression is that of a slowed down, even arrested time, accompanied by the slowing down of thought and motor skills, and the collapse of the past–present–future perspective. In this state of psychic near-death, the ordinary temporality of human life is seriously disturbed, and Fédida specifies that "depression is indeed *a human disease of time* that affects representation and action, the potentialities of language, as well as communication with others" (p. 22, italics added). Consequently, it goes without saying that it is not a question of forcing an either/or choice between the temporal and the other metapsychological points of view, since the temporal dimension is part and parcel of the possibility of representation and communication. I find another support in Fédida's thinking when he writes that "the psychopathology of time in depressed states concerns [...] both the body of action and intersubjective communication" (p. 23).

Depression and the unpast

In my previous work on psychic temporality (Scarfone, 2015), I have tried to show that in our clinical experience with various psychopathological forms we always encounter a nucleus of "actual time", a form of time that I also proposed to call "the *unpast*" in order to emphasize both its character of *arrested time* and of *impasse*. The disorder of temporality in depression seems to me to egregiously illustrate this form of time, revealed as it is by the erasure of psychic life described by Fédida. Admittedly, depressive immobilization does not erase all temporality, but it does highlight the experience of a dead-end in time, a "time that does not pass", as Pontalis (1997) wrote.

In my use of the term "actual" one can easily recognize the nosographic category of "actual neuroses" posited by Freud by contrast with the psychoneuroses.[1] In the Freudian classification, actual neuroses were initially two: anxiety neurosis and neurasthenia; later he added hypochondria. For us analysts, it matters that, contrary to diagnostic manuals such as the DSM, it is not so much the signs and symptoms – identified by the clinical *gaze* – but rather the challenge that these states pose to our *listening* that gives us the key to their differentiation. Psychoanalytic listening, in fact, helps us detect the specific metapsychological features of actual neuroses: from the *dynamic* point of view, the erasing of psychoneurotic conflictuality; from the *topical* point of view, the thinness if not the non-existence of the mediating function of the pre-conscious – namely a language without metaphors, without slips, without double meanings – and the impoverishment of the oneiric life; from the *economic* point of view, the tendency to motor discharge or else to a discharge that Freud called "secretory", that is to say, occurring inside the body, which contributes to somatizations. As Michel de M'Uzan indicated, even sexual activity in these cases takes on the value of a mere discharge of tension (de M'Uzan, 1994). If we now look at the *temporal* point of view, we first notice a linearization of time, that is, the absence of the complex, *après-coup* time loops observable in psychoneurotic organizations. Moreover, in depression, time itself seems seriously slowed down if not arrested, sometimes fixated on opaque elements of previous history – something that often induces clinicians to invoke traumatic, organic or even genetic factors. The result of this arrested time is that the experience is always "present", or better: "actual", in the literal sense of Freud's adjective "*aktual*" in "*Aktualneurosen*", i.e . *presently active* with no apparent internal conflict or phantasmatic template. This means that the historical roots of the problem are not easily retrievable, and it is therefore difficult to relegate such "present" experience to the past. This makes me suggest that actual time, or the *unpast,* is the form of time pertaining to the dark core of psychic life.

From a nosographic point of view, the Paris School of Psychosomatics has based itself on Freud's metapsychology to highlight what were dubbed "operative states" (*états opératoires*) and the essential depression mentioned earlier. A "depression without an object", essential depression is radically different from melancholic depression since it does not include the classic psychic symptoms of the latter, such as self-reproach and self-despising that follow the incorporation of the lost object. I will not linger here on the details of essential depression nor on its intimate relationship with operative states, of which one can find masterful descriptions in Marty and de M'Uzan (1963). However, I would like to propose that, just as there exists a nucleus of actual neurosis at the heart of the best-mentalized psychoneuroses (Freud 1915–1917, p. 390), so at the heart of all depressions, whatever the degree of mentalization, there exists a nucleus of essential depression, a nucleus which I would also call *actual* in the sense described above. When this actual core of depression cannot be shrouded in an effective psychical coating,[2] the temporal disorganization typical of all depressions ensues in variable forms and degrees.

A caveat is in order here, as the surface clinical phenomena may be misleading. Melancholia, indeed, seems to be well anchored in the past while essential depression is stuck in the present. Except that even in melancholia the " past" has invaded the present and is experienced in the " actual" mode; as for the " present" of essential depression, it expresses in fact a total lack of historical perspective, hence it is not the " present" in the ordinary sense of a time swiftly flowing toward the past and open to the advent of the future.

However, it is true that a measure of psychical shrouding *is* present in melancholia, as manifested by fantasies of incorporation and the preeminence of guilt delusions, making for a very different picture than that of essential depression where no such psychical coating can be found. Still, the actual core is present in melancholia just as well, so one could say that essential (or actual) depression is to melancholia what anxiety neurosis is to hysteria.

The presence of this obscure actual core is not at all surprising once one realizes that the core-to-coating relationship – which is tacitly present within all psychopathological entities and current psychic phenomena – can therefore be expected in depression as well. One can indeed detect in Freud's writings a recurrent pattern, superimposable on the model of the relationship we have just evoked between actual neuroses and psychoneuroses. Thus, very early on, in his *Studies on Hysteria*, Freud posited the existence of a traumatic core lodged beneath the complex strata of hysterical representations; in *The Interpretation of Dreams*, he twice emphasized the existence of a navel at the heart of every dream, a navel which, being linked to the unknown, prevents a complete analysis of the dream. In the same way, one can think of the *Unheimlich* core at the heart of the familiar, which only emerges in particular situations.[3] The most general model of this relation between a core and its coating is to be found in the 1895 *Project*, where Freud described a "perceptual complex" or "complex of the fellow human being", consisting of an understandable part (dubbed "predicate" or " attributes") and enshrouding an incomprehensible nucleus that evades judgement and which he dubbed *the Thing (das Ding)* (Freud, 1895, p. 331, 334). A similar (core/coating) pattern can be found in the works of other authors: the Real at the heart of reality but radically distinct from it (Lacan); the sexual enigma at the heart of the compromised message from adult to infant (Laplanche); the traces of a collapse that has already occurred, but was not recorded and is now apprehended as lying ahead (Winnicott, 1963).

By situating essential depression as the actual nucleus at the center of all depression, I am therefore subscribing to the Freudian logic according to which, indeed, the psychic is a " dressing" of the actual. A coating made of representations that allows for the elaboration of a story, even if the actual core itself shall always escape the passage of time.

The test of the psychic facts

The question is now to verify if this general model fits with the clinical facts. What does it mean, clinically, to say that any form of clinical depression contains a kernel of essential depression, that is to say, an actual core without representations, without fantasy of incorporation of the lost object? First, let us note that this is completely congruent with what I quoted at the beginning from Fédida's work where depression is conceived of as the erasure of psychic life itself. Conversely, as already indicated, it also allows us to conceive of melancholic phenomenology as the psychic envelope of an actual depressive core. A fragile envelope, to be sure, presumably a last resort, an emergency measure when the psyche faces severe loss.

Nicolas Abraham (1978) once suggested that the melancholic subject has been incapable of a true *process* of introjection, substituted with a *fantasy* of incorporation. The capacity to fantasize incorporation is certainly preferable to a total psychic collapse, but the fact remains that the ghost – or the shadow – of the incorporated object which has invaded the ego is itself covered by a layer of painful self-accusations that can lead to self-annihilation. What is thus draped in a delusion is an unthinkable loss, a loss of psychic substance, as it were, that the more psychical melancholic layer is trying to make up for. Melancholia therefore appears indeed as a mentalized version of depression, yet without implying a difference in nature as to the fundamental phenomenon. It does not differ either, in terms of mentalization, from the manic reaction, except by its reversed polarity.

Heeding the actual kernel within the more elaborate clinical picture of melancholia indicates to us, firstly, that there is no break, but continuity in the conception of the various depressive modalities; secondly, it reminds us that clinical reality does not let itself be locked in watertight compartments. Continuity in fact admits intermediate forms which, far from being fixed entities, allow us to envisage possible movements of mentalization and elaboration as I hope to now show.

Elvira

Elvira is a patient I have written about in an older paper (Scarfone, 1990). She was referred to me because, several months after the death of her mother (of whom she was the only child), she was still in a state of prostration, with psychomotor retardation, severe anorexia and significant weight loss, though without any spectacular self-reproach or suicidal ideation; an array of symptoms that had not responded to various antidepressants.

During our first meetings I learned from Elvira that her mother lived in an apartment just above hers and came down every morning to look after the children when she and her husband were at work. One morning, however, on the day after Elvira and her mother had fiercely quarreled (as sometimes happened), the mother didn't come down, which at first made Elvira think that she was still angry with her; but as it was getting late, she went upstairs hoping to make peace with her mother and have her come and stay with the children as usual. She rang and rang and finally resolved to use her key to her mother's apartment, only to find her lying dead in her bed.

Apart from the scene of this discovery, everything in Elvira's memory became blurred. She had, however, the hazy memory of having lost control and having frantically punched her mother's dead body. She must have hit herself too, she said, because she later found her own body covered in bruises. After which she fell into a deep state of depression.

During our sessions, it was soon possible for Elvira to speak in more detail about what made her lose her appetite completely. "It is", she said, "because of a bad taste in my mouth. The taste of cadaver". From there, we went on to explore Elvira's complicated relationship to her mother, their repeated scrambles and reconciliations, and began putting into words the fantasy of cannibalistic incorporation clearly suggested by the "taste of cadaver" at the root of her inappetence. Elvira started eating again and our sessions became host to the elaboration of the painful process of grieving her loss, a process that had been blocked until then.

After six months of this twice-a-week, face-to-face analytical work, Elvira seemed to have completely come out of her depression; she had regained her energy and resumed all her activities. Everything was going well, at least on the surface. The sessions with me, to which Elvira was very assiduous, had however become increasingly dull, full of banal anecdotes about her daily activities or the weather ... This lasted another six months, before, bored and somewhat exasperated, I dared put to her the idea that since everything seemed to be back to normal, we could envisage an end to our meetings at some point in the near future.

Elvira's reaction was massive: she, who seemed to come to our sessions only routinely, felt a painful sense of abandonment, not understanding at all that I was thinking of ending her treatment. Following which, not only did we continue our work together, but after the summer vacations Elvira came back having made an important discovery. While visiting her mother's apartment with a friend, she stumbled upon a photograph of her early childhood. In the photo, which she brought and showed me, she is held at arm's length by a nun. In the room around them, other nuns are busy with other children placed in small metallic cribs. To her puzzled friend Elvira suddenly declared, as if in a state of trance: "That's me, I'm in an orphanage; I stayed there until I was one year old!" Elvira had no idea where this information came from; the words, she says, just came out of her mouth as if under pressure.

The patient then said that the photo in question was in fact one she had often seen among her mother's things, but that when she had asked questions about it, she only got evasive answers. Now, thanks to this same photograph, Elvira felt confident she could reconstruct at least part of her early history. After further inquiries, she found that, unlike what the picture suggested, she was not an orphan whom her mother would have adopted. More probably, she thought, her mother had to temporarily "place" her in the institution at the age of six months to protect her from a violent psychotic father. The family photo album – which tracked the child's development until she was about six months old and then resumed, showing her after her first birthday, hence leaving a six month blank – fitted well indeed with the reconstructed timeline of the events.

By going back to Elvira's case I wished to illustrate how, after evoking the possible end of the treatment, her discovery of the photo, and the recon-struction of an early abandonment that ensued, gave her access to a pain even deeper than the one caused by the recent loss of her mother. Through the après-coup reverberation between two distant periods of her life that was allowed by the analytic work, we were able to touch on a primordial, poorly mentalized layer of depression. The lack of memories about this early period had resulted – as we were now able to understand – in repetitions in action that had occurred throughout her childhood. Such as, for instance, young Elvira's hitherto inexplicable ritual of packing her bundle every Sunday and announcing that she was leaving home (she was between five and ten years old), forcing her mother to go looking for her in the neighborhood! Elvira now thought that she was thus unknowingly and compulsively repeating the trauma of separation followed by the joy of retrieval.

In the sessions that followed her important discovery, Elvira decided to start using the couch, but she immediately found it unbearable not being able to see me. So I offered her to move my chair so that I could stay in her field of vision. This clearly comforted her, for she then cowered on the couch in the fetal position and started sobbing without restraint. The sobbing went on for much of the next few weeks. The work of grieving had resumed, at a level and with an intensity that I could not have suspected. In retrospect, it looks as if the interpretation of oral incorporation in our first series of encounters had, so to speak, scraped a first psychic layer – the one I described as quasi-melancholic – thus unintentionally opening the way to a deeper and more essential depressive core. Fortunately for Elvira, who was a professional photographer, her interest in pictures had provided an external representational support thanks to which it was possible for her to construct what was perhaps a personal myth, but one that she believed told the true story of her object-loss. A loss that had happened in a too early period to be registered as a memory, and which the recent death of the mother had brought into the "actual" a-historic present. Within the framework of the transferential scene, she was allowed to formulate her long and painful complaint about abandonment at a young age and to put it, for the first time, "into the past tense", as Winnicott (1963) would say, making it a narrative rather than a source of repetition in action.

Closing remarks

With the example of Elvira I tried to illustrate how the psychotherapy of the depressive states navigates along a temporal axis, between the two poles of a basic psychic structuring which I believe is common to all mental formations, normal or pathological: an "actual" pole, not psychically representable, and a properly psychic pole covering, with varied results, that "actual" pole, and allowing for the introduction of chronological time, hence the construction of a past.

In the case of Elvira, the initial clinical tableau was one of quasi-melancholia, as attested by the fantasy of oral incorporation of the mother's corpse. The resolution of this episode gave way to a kind of abrasion of the psychic layer and the emergence of a more opaque core, whose previous inaccessibility had given the sessions with Elvira their "operative" and boring aspect. After the first six months, she was apparently no longer depressed, but her psyche had been confined to the banality of everyday life. My countertransferential blunder, however, opened up something even deeper and more painful; something which had not yet found a psychic terrain where fantasy could play its part. The rediscovery of a photograph gave Elvira an external prop on which to weave a plausible story, allowing her to "put into the past tense" the hitherto *unpast* drama of her loss of object.

In another case, which I cannot report here for confidentiality's sake, actual states of panic alternating with severe, non-melancholic depression found their psychic shroud through the temporary formation of an hypochondriac fantasy. The analysis of this hypochondria opened the road to reaching a kernel of affect unheard of until that moment. Though Freud considered hypochondria an outright actual neurosis, its occurrence during treatment seems an interesting event in that it indicates a certain fluidity, even a gradation, between the more discrete clinical forms of actual neuroses and psychoneuroses. In the case in question, the analytic process, with the transferential relationship at its center, allowed for the constitution of an intermediate psychic layer more likely to enshroud the dark "actual" core within a usable representational mantle.

Notes

1 Freud distinguished from early on between actual neuroses and the psychoneuroses of defence, as is noticeable in various papers in Volume 3 of the Standard Edition; he discussed them more at length in the Introductory lectures (Freud, 1915–17, pp. 385–390).
2 The notion of "psychical coating" is used by Freud in various texts to describe the relationship between the representational aspect, in hysterical symptoms for instance, and the "actual" core. A clear example is in the analysis of Dora (Freud, 1905, p. 84 and 99n2).
3 More on this aspect in (Scarfone, 2015 p. 122 ff).

References

Abraham, N. (1978). *Introjecter, incorporer: deuil ou mélancolie in L'écorce et le noyau*. Paris: Aubier.
Bergson, H. (1895). *Matière et mémoire*. Paris: PUF, "Quadrige".
De M'Uzan, M. (1994). Slaves of quantity. *Psychoanalytic Quarterly*, LXXII, 2003, 711–725.
Fédida, P. (2001). *Des bienfaits de la dépression*. Paris: Odile Jacob.
Freud, S. (1895). Project for a scientific psychology. *Standard Edition of the Complete Works of Sigmund Freud* (hereafter: *S.E.*) I. London: The Hogarth Press and The Institute of Psychoanalysis, pp. 283–397.
Freud, S. (1905). Fragment of an analysis of a case of hysteria. *S.E.* 7, pp. 7–122.
Freud, S. (1915–17). Introductory lectures on psychoanalysis (Part III). *S.E.* 14, pp. 385–390.

Freud, S. (1933). New introductory lessons on psychoanalysis. *S.E.* 22, pp. 74.

Marty, P. (1968). La dépression essentielle. *Revue française de psychanalyse*, XXXII(1), 595–598.

Marty, P. & de M'Uzan, M. (1963). La pensée opératoire. *Revue Française de Psychanalyse*, XXVII, special issue, 345–356.

Pontalis, J-B. (1997). *Ce temps qui ne passe pas*. Paris: Gallimard, coll. "Tracés".

Scarfone, D. (1990). Jardins de pierres. *"L'épreuve du temps": Nouvelle revue de psychanalyse*, 41, 279–289.

Scarfone, D. (2006). A matter of time: Actual time and the production of the past. *The Psychoanalytic Quarterly*, LXXV, 807–833.

Scarfone, D. (2015). *The unpast: The actual unconscious*. New York: The Unconscious in Translation.

Winnicott, D. W. (1963). *Fear of breakdown: Psychoanalytic explorations*. Cambridge, MA: Harvard University Press, 1989, pp. 87–95.

4 The invisible depression

Nicolas de Coulon

The very question of the psychoanalytic approach to depression is likely to rekindle clinicians' interest in a condition that has often been left to the care of the psychiatrist. Certain elements of seriousness contribute to this state of affairs, in particular when the phenomena of sideration predominate with the sensation of an ineluctable slope leading to death. As Pierre Fédida (Fédida, 2001) puts it: "the intuition of the annihilation of all psychic life comes to accredit the belief that depression would only be a kind of biological or neurobiological illness requiring the sole recourse to antidepressant drugs". Psychoanalysis makes it possible to question the psychopathological foundations as well as the psychotherapeutic handling of it by focusing on what we can consider as the recognition of a work of the negative within the psychic life itself.

For all these reasons, this chapter will be particularly interested in the submerged part of the depressive iceberg, the invisible components of depression. This is not the easiest part to discuss when it comes to conducting clinical research, with its need to consider marks, signalling points that identify the intensity of the depressive disorder in a sufficiently visible way. Indeed, it is often only at this price that a major contribution of psychoanalytic therapies for depression can be recognised and accepted by the scientific world. However, I believe that it is necessary to keep in touch with what is the heart of our discipline, namely the unconscious and its indirect manifestations. In this sense, it is not only the negative mood of the patients that is at stake but also the internal negative underlying the depressive variations. I could therefore just as easily have titled the present chapter as follows: the conditions of psychoanalytic visibility of depression or even the work of the negative in depression.

The first part will be devoted to a discussion of the rich and controversial notion of unconscious affect, while the second part will re-evaluate the importance of depression in the transference (transference depression), which arises during the psychoanalytic treatment. One of the conclusions will probably be read as we go along, since it concerns a rehabilitation of depression, such as can be found both in Melanie Klein's notion of the depressive position, and in Pierre Fédida's proposition, which stresses the importance of access to depressivity – in short, what could be described in terms of depressive capacity, a quality that must be recovered in order to overcome existential and psychological crises.

DOI: 10.4324/9781003279297-4

Unconscious affect

Affect and its manifestations, as well as its function in the cure, remained for a long time ignored in metapsychological thinking. In particular, French psycho-analysis was mainly concerned with representation and the signifier, for example in a Lacanian perspective. It was André Green who put affect back at the centre of reflections in his report to the congress of French-speaking psychoanalysts (Green, 1970). This text became a book that made a name for itself, "Le discours vivant" (Green, 1973). Since then, it has been easier for us to follow what, in psychoanalytic practice, takes into account the embodiment of the language in bodily and affective experience. It is thus a question of restoring the importance of the "affect–representative", to use the Freudian formulation which underlines an important function of affect, that of *"representance"*, which we can describe as messenger within the psyche and in inter-psychic communication, between self and other, between subject and object. As the title of a well-known book suggests, *Descartes' error: Emotion, Reason and the Human Brain* (Damasio, 1994), this concern joins with the work of biologists, ethnologists, neuroscientists and early childhood clinicians while facilitating our dialogue with them.

The question of the unconscious dimension of affect is of particular interest to psychoanalysts. It should be recalled that affect is generally recognised as belonging rather to consciousness, allowing us to rehabilitate the latter (Solms & Panksepp, 2015), even among psychoanalysts. In contrast, Freud had pro-posed a notion that has already given rise to many contradictory opinions, that of *unconscious affect*. We remember that it was about inferring a feeling about a major effect in the lives of patients, for example to understand the negative therapeutic reaction in relation to the unconscious feeling of guilt and the need for punishment, opening up what we can call the problem of masochism (Freud, 1924c).

The discussion on this subject is not very simple and I will sketch it out in broad strokes. In the Freudian proposal, an unconscious affect can only be identified from its effects: in the manifestations that cannot be understood without a certain number of hypotheses, such as the identification of the actions of a guilty person who ignores himself, who moreover seeks to be punished, who prefers pain to pleasure (masochism), who wants to remain sick rather than to get better. Naturally, in order to observe these mechan-isms, we are more at ease in the psychoanalyst's laboratory, i.e. its chair and couch setting, than in that of the neuroscientist. We also need a certain familiarity with the clinical work of the negative, the work that takes into consideration elements that are not only latent, but hidden, inverted, on the side of absence or emptiness. All this requires reference to the framework of the second Freudian metapsychology, the framework that allows the exten-sion of our cures to borderline states, to identity–narcissistic sufferings, as we can call them, following René Roussillon.

It is in fact from the latter author that I borrow part of this comment. In an article on affect, Roussillon (2005) goes back to the Freudian text that could be considered as a precursor of a neuro-psychoanalytic perspective, *Inhibition, Symptom and Anxiety* (Freud, 1926), by underlining that affect is a biological necessity within the framework of the danger situation. In this, Freud follows Darwin who said that the emotional response corresponds to a set of coherent somatic reactions, organised in relation to a particular situation and involving an action. From this mobilisation of the body, we can follow the path of information given to the psyche about biological affective processes. These messages would be addressed both internally to the subject itself and externally to others in the relationship with the primary object, thus becoming what Roussillon calls a primary animal language. In this sense, affect is either a signal or a message, what Freud calls a representative. This explains why psychoanalysts are more familiar with the terminology of representative–affect than with more biologising or computational vocabularies.

The construction of the affect

Classically, it is the representative–representation that is repressed, as we well know, but there is nothing to prevent us from thinking that the organisation of the associative network of somatic connections leading to a recognisable emotion can remain, in whole or in part, unconscious. Thus, we can consider that the psychic representation of the affect coming from the body is constructed, that it is composed. This is already apparent when we try to distinguish the so-called primary forms of affect (joy, sadness, disgust, fear) from the more complex so-called secondary forms (shame, guilt, disappointment, etc.). We would perhaps tend to consider the immediacy of the feeling expressed or shown as a sort of reflex arc that imposes it as a primary, unbreakable evidence. However, even neuroscientific discoveries do not point in this direction. This construction of affect may also imply taking into account a characteristic that is usually left out in measures of feeling, namely the temporal dimension: indeed, the short-circuit model is not totally applicable. Even if it is subject to more or less rapid variations, the affect takes a certain amount of time to settle, to organise itself and to evolve before disappearing or giving way to another feeling. Moreover, the progressive establishment of the affective palette and its composition obviously depend on the characteristics of the primary environment and more specifically on the response of the object. Thus, joy can be brief, but shame and guilt can last. This is also the case of depression, defined as a complex emotion, gathering several basic affects.

Therefore, we could consider depression as a complicated, constructed, form of sadness. It requires the consideration of temporal evolution, which is confirmed both by clinical observation and by the more theoretical understanding of *Mourning and Melancholia* (Freud, 1917). For Freud, the quality of affect is related to its temporality, in particular its duration. It is therefore more difficult to measure than its intensity, its quantitative value (the quantum of affect). It is interesting to note that this charge and duration are underlined by the psychoanalytic notion of work, dream work, mourning work or work of melancholia. The psychotherapy of the depressed state could well be called depression work, or if one prefers a more dynamic idea, depression crossing.

These metapsychological considerations suggest the participation of the unconscious in the making of affect and its expression. As a result, we cannot be satisfied with too basic definitions of the division between a representation that could be repressed and an affect that could not be repressed, which would always be completely conscious. The complexity of the psyche comes into play again.

Variations in visibility

There is no shortage of other arguments about the invisibility of affect, when we consider its unconscious properties in more detail. For example, in constraint neurosis, there is a particularly marked disconnection between affect and representation. The representation remains, devoid of the affect that classically comes to be displaced on another image. Under these conditions, is the affect really only displaced, can it not be repressed, at least in part? Is it not the same for certain paths of internal derivation leading to somatisation and opening the field of the psychosomatic clinic? The very notion of repression of affect most often indicates a mixed mechanism, both conscious and unconscious. This presupposes that we clarify what we mean by repression in this type of situation because the line of thought obviously concerns the second topical approach, as we have already mentioned, when the development of repression is complicated by the mechanisms of denial and splitting.

It would thus be a question of taking into consideration a more psycho-pathological dimension. For certain individuals, at certain moments in their trajectory, the ways of representing and perhaps even perceiving the affect are modified and disturbed. The risk of overflow is so great that the ego can come to defend itself by insensitivity or even inaffectivity, as we have just mentioned for the constraint neurosis. There would be much to say on the same problem in the borderline states. To remain brief, we know that the emotional response can be translated into action, transformed into acting (in or out), through movement. The affect may be intense, even explosive, but it is disqualified, in the sense of an expression that is much more quantitative than qualitative, and not very differentiated. It is highly probable that the knotting between the affective discharge and the acting out takes place, here too, at an unconscious level. On this subject, we can keep the expression of Dominique Scarfone (2020) who speaks of a "psychic coating" bringing into play both the affective elements and the displacement of representations. Moreover, the temporal and topical intertwining refers us to the original aspects and the conditions of construction of the early relationship to the parents, to the mother.

With the clinic of early trauma, we should be able to explore some of the basic conditions of the composition of affect. A patient, Mrs. P., begins her psychoanalysis after a period of psychotherapy in which she was able to metabolise the aftermath of a painful divorce. For a long time, the symptoms concern her anxiety states and the obsessive mechanisms that allow her to organise her work despite the wound of this rupture. Finally, depressive affects arise and depression sets in. The loss of objects goes back several years, but we can then observe a Winnicottian phenomenon: it is the fear of breakdown which becomes the central element of the analytical treatment but which forces us to go back to Mrs. P.'s childhood. While her usual version described a sometimes exaggerated presence of the mother, a recent revelation of the latter mentions an absence, an early separation, due to an illness of this mother of which the patient had kept no memory. In retrospect, we can think that the melancholic elements were not accessible to Mrs. P, nor to her nor to me for that matter, at the beginning of the face-to-face and even of the analytic treatment. The depression was invisible. This observation ties in with another proposal, that of Marianne Leuzinger (Leuzinger-Bohleber, 2015), which concerns the traumatic hypothesis. This was already present in Freud (Freud, 1924c): "states of affect are incorporated into the life of the soul as precipitates of very old traumatic lived experiences and are evoked in similar situations as mnemonic symbols".

In this way, we highlight the double dimension of depressive affects, both conscious and unconscious, which justifies the intervention of the psychoanalyst in the field of depression and his interest in what is called *the dark side* in this book on depressive states. It is not only a question of black versus white, of sadness versus joy, but of what is hidden and withdrawn – in a word, of the importance of the work of the negative in psychoanalysis. Depressive affect can be invisible, concealed, counter-invested, split off, denied and it is up to the clinician to contribute to its recognition.

Depression in the transference

As we have just seen, the conditions of visibility of depression are not always identical. Another example specific to the psychoanalytic field could obey another denomination, formerly known even in the related field of psychiatry under the name of "masked" depression. This is transference depression, described mainly by André Green (Green, 1980) in his beautiful text on "the Dead Mother".

In the clinical description, the patient has no memory or awareness of what happened early on. This can only be reconstructed in the treatment in the form of a *revelation in the transference*. We can describe it as follows: despite the evocative title, the mother is not really dead, she has not even disappeared momentarily as in real separations, inflicted for a more or less long time. In fact, she was no longer emotionally present for her child for a certain period of time. She is emotionally absent. It is therefore a question of a maternal affective withdrawal in early childhood, a withdrawal that occurs following an intense upheaval in the mother, often a bereavement that strikes her. When the analysand consults, it is usually for repeated failures in his or her love life. It is necessary to emphasise this point, because in this case the patient does not come for help because of sad prostration. The patient does not usually present a depressive display, neither acute nor chronic. However, it is a depression that qualifies the disorder, an *invisible depression*. Indeed, just because a patient does not, at first sight, present a depressed state does not mean that the question of depression does not arise. In particular, we must consider the notion evoked by Green as a thread towards the discovery of the complex, namely the procession of depressive affects that emerge in the treatment itself after some time, perhaps even after several months or years. The patient is not depressed, he/she gets depressed during the psychoanalytic process. By analogy with the notion of transference neurosis, Green speaks of transference depression, of a transferential movement that will have to be interpreted – which is not necessarily very simple – after having identified and detailed with the patient what it is about. Most often, the depression can be contained within the setting of the sessions, not appearing outside or in daily life. It is especially with the psychoanalyst that the patient is depressed and communicates negative feelings. Gradually, representations arise around the famous "dead mother" complex, moments of childhood when the mother was unavailable, herself captive of a mourning. This could not make sense in the experience of the child, who no longer received the quality care he or she had obtained up to that point. This lack, this emotional absence will gradually become traumatic, while being encapsulated in the psyche, causing more relational disorders than mood disorders. On rare occasions, the melancholic side may spill over outside the sessions and take on clinical significance. When the depression manifests itself and can be addressed in the treatment, it becomes an important turning point in the analysis. From negative, it becomes positive!

We can again follow the emergence of particular and psychoanalytically significant conditions of visibility. Other more direct observers might compare the effects of a child's depression with that of an adult. It is perhaps not very surprising that emotional difficulties in childhood are transformed in many ways into what will become adult suffering. André Green and other authors (Bergeret, 1980) identify and follow them in what we can consider as borderline pathologies or borderline states. Depression would then be part of the structure, disappearing behind it and only revealing itself when the psychoanalytical conditions are met.

In this way, the modes of appearance of an invisible depression bring us back to Winnicott and his conceptions (Winnicott, 1954) who speaks of thawing. The earliest pathological elements would be caught in a frozen envelope and only the establishment of the necessary trust could allow them to thaw, typically the establishment of a good enough transferential relationship. The symptomatic outbreak of depressive affects, the more or less clinically perceptible depression, thus becomes a way of accessing them emotionally before being able to figure them out and then represent them.

A patient had undertaken analysis to get rid of a compulsion that repeatedly led him to enter into relationships that proved unsatisfactory and led to break-ups. The rest of his life worked fairly well and he was successful in his career. On the face of it, his childhood had been relatively happy except for a disagreement with an overbearing father who was hard on him, causing him to reject the father. The tender relationship with the mother had also been abruptly interrupted by this father in the oedipal period and had contributed to the resentment just mentioned. The patient remembered having to fend for himself somewhat alone, without support from that point on, which contributed to his isolation and a deficit in his relationships. The mother had died a few years before our psychoanalysis began. In our sessions, the patient's mood was initially quite jovial and he spoke without too much difficulty, even about current and past disappointments. We had analysed the oedipal period extensively and the scene we have just mentioned, which took the form of a ban on entering the parents' bedroom. It was only after more than two years of analysis that the patient began to feel less dynamic and cheerful. A certain dissatisfaction arose in the transference which could at first be interpreted in the paternal register. In spite of this, the sadness affects persisted without preventing the patient from living his life, but the climate of the sessions became heavy. The analysis of the maternal transference yielded few results until, following a long holiday by the analyst, the patient felt really worse. He then began to question his father, with whom he had in the meantime resumed contact, and learned that his mother's illness, which he vaguely remembered, and which had kept her bedridden for several weeks, was in fact a depression. We were thus able to reconstruct the story. When he was not even two years old, his mummy had lost her mother suddenly, which had made her melancholic and unavailable to her child for several months. The patient had no memory of this. It was a *dead mother* in the sense of André Green. The transference depression had thus gradually set in. It was only through a transferential reaction around the holidays, accompanied by a family revelation, that it was possible to really analyse the transference depression. Without going into detail, we can say that the patient's affects were able to emerge from the depressive envelope and that the analysis then developed favourably.

In other words, the passage through the transference depression follows a pattern that we find quite often in analytic cures. At the beginning, the psychic elements are relatively mobile and the symptoms mild. Then comes a phase in which the painful, static and fixed components typical of depression develop, with the characteristic that the analyst becomes the central object of the negativity. If the treatment evolves favourably, we witness the return of a more easily analysable mobility which is inscribed in the dynamics of the transference and which will allow a liquidation, at least partial, of the depressive core.

The benefits of depression

Clearly, what is most important in clinical depression is the psychological pain. This is probably why it is difficult to envisage another invisible aspect, the good side of depression, what Pierre Fédida (2001) calls the benefits.

Could it be that this aspect is made imperceptible in the psychiatric care of depressed patients? As we have just seen, there is a wide range of differences between, on the one hand, melancholia as an illness linked to death (or even to the death drive), and on the other hand, an invisible wound that can only manifest itself under certain good enough psychotherapeutic conditions. This is why the range of depressive illness should not make us forget the properly psychic and human component put at the service of an internal potentiality. For Melanie Klein (1935), depression is already a normal process! It is a question, for the baby, of finding the way to integrate the good sides of the object with the bad ones, to link the contradictory fantasies and the opposite feelings that it encounters inside itself and in its relationship to primary objects. Subsequently, this psychoanalytic theorist will develop the idea not of an illness but of a stage, *the depressive position*, which is very important in any psychic evolution but also in all psychotherapeutic cures.

In our idea, it would be a sort of interweavement necessary to the psychological balance, carried out by the unconscious ego, at the crossroads between affects and representations. It is this idea that Pierre Fédida takes up when he distinguishes depressive capacity from pathological depression. For him, symptomatic movements should be followed with great precision, for example by distinguishing sadness as a return to movement from melancholic immobility. He goes even further with his notion of *depressivity* as a capacity for openness/closure to contact with the other, to rhythm, to resonance and to the internal regulation of excitations. In short, it could be put in correspondence with the Freudian notion of the protective shield, provided that it is not only thought of as a maternal function, but also as a simultaneous production of the baby itself. The latter would thus protect oneself from too strong external loads, from the brutality of the changes brought about by the external world. It is the construction of subjectivity that is at stake and in this sense, depressivity is to be placed on the side of Winnicottian creativity and therefore of transitional phenomena.

Another parallel can be drawn with the more general occurrence of psychological crises (de Coulon, 2021), those which plunge the subject into an acute malaise, the foundations of which remain incomprehensible at first. In these cases, the malaise is not necessarily depressive, but the symptomatology is noisy. It is only in a second phase that it is possible to detect the evolutionary potential, to see clearly, to keep our metaphor around the visible and the invisible.

Finally, we could ask ourselves if this *negative of depression*, its invisibility, does not in some way represent a therapeutic opportunity provided by depression. Starting from the idea that it was necessary to take an interest in the hidden, invisible aspects of depression, we would have identified some of the internal resources hidden by the negative terminology. We could therefore retain "a good use of depression as a 'negative process' allowing the subject to protect himself against the always possible danger of melancholic annihilation" (Roudinesco, 2001). The acceptance of psychic pain and its transformation are part of the psychoanalytic process, an additional opportunity to grasp the unconscious motions, and therefore invisible, in our cures.

References

Bergeret, J. (1980). *La dépression et les états-limites.* Paris: Payot.

Damasio, A. R. (1994). *Descartes' error, emotion, reason and the human brain*, Ed. A. Grosset. New York, NY: Putnam Books.

De Coulon, N. (2021). *La crise, stratégies d'intervention thérapeutique en psychiatrie.* Lausanne: Antipodes.

Fédida, P. (2001). *Des bienfaits de la dépression, éloge de la psychothérapie.* Paris: Éditions Odile Jacob.

Freud, S. (1917). *Deuil et mélancolie, OCF-P*, vol. XIII. Paris: PUF.

Freud, S. (1924c). *Le problème économique du masochisme, OCF-P*, XVII, p. 21. Paris: PUF.

Freud, S. (1926). *Inhibition, symptôme et angoisse, OCF-P*, XVII. Paris: PUF.

Green, A. (1970). *L'affect.* Paris: PUF.

Green, A. (1973). *Le discours vivant.* Paris: PUF.

Green, A. (1980). *La mère morte, in Narcissisme de vie, Narcissisme de mort.* Paris: PUF.

Klein, M. (1935). A contribution to the psychogenesis of manic-depressive states. *International Journal of Psychoanalysis*, 16, 145–174.

Leuzinger-Bohleber, M. (2015). Working with severely traumatized, chronically depressed analysands. *International Journal of Psychoanalysis*, 96, 611–636.

Roudinesco, E. (2001). *Du bon usage de la dépression*, article de présentation du livre cité de Pierre Fédida dans Le Monde des Livres, 9 February 2001.

Roussillon, R. (2005). *Affect inconscient, affect-passion et affect-signal. Monographies de psychanalyse, l'affect.* Paris: PUF.

Scarfone, D. (2023). Clinical and conceptual psychoanalytical approaches to depression and trauma, Chapter 3, this volume.

Solms, M., & Panksepp, J. (2015). Why depression feels bad. In: C. H. Ashton & E. K. Perry (Eds.), *New horizons in the neuroscience of conscious.* Amsterdam: John Benjamins.

Winnicott, D. W. (1954). Metapsychological and clinical aspects of regression within the psycho-analytical set-up. In: *Through paediatrics to psycho-analysis.* London: Hogarth Press (1987); in French: *Les aspects métapsychologique que et clinique de la régression au sein de la situation analytique in de la Pédiatrie à la psychanalyse.* Paris: Payot (trad. 1969).

5 The denied object of melancholy

J. C. Rolland

Freudian metapsychology is a strong heritage left by the founder that needs to be updated in the light of the deepening of analytic practice. Analytic practice has changed a lot since Freud, more than we think and say, especially with regard to listening and the technique of interpretation, so in fact with regard to the evaluation of the relations of language and the word to the unconscious.

Metapsychological thinking is first of all a method of thinking: its constructions are born in the inner discourse of the analyst in contact with the associative discourse of the patient and they capture unconscious formations that manifest themselves *in statu nascendi*; unconscious formations always keep a distance from the traces of the real history, retaining only the pulsional underpinning. These constructions, once assembled, serve as a compass to listen to the psychic forces at work, for discerning the material, made of words and images, that make up the patient's psyche; it is a speculative, visionary thought.

The particularity of the depressive state is that it is an "alienating" illness but also a (salutary) defence against deeper and silent suffering; it calls for help from the patient, always coupled with a determination (not a will) not to be cured. Would this also be the case with autoimmune diseases? The patient with depression opposes his treatment with a mysterious and powerful resistance in which one suspects either a method of survival or a source of pleasure, an enjoyment. The depressive state thus always includes a division of the being, one fraction of it wants, another refuses; each of the parts taking control of the consciousness and the psychomotor apparatus, or personifying itself more or less in a fraction of one's ego, barely discernible from one's object. In every patient with depression, there is thus partly an active avoidance of any care, and more broadly of any interference by the other, an avoidance that necessarily hinders the psychotherapeutic process and in which the patient actively cooperates by forbidding or dissuading the analyst from approaching him or her.

The internal object to which the depressive clings is his idol. The symbol of this clinging is the *Noli me tangere* uttered by Christ to Mary Magdalene at the end of his resurrection on the grounds that "he has not yet ascended to the father and that only there, in his absence, will he become accessible to the

DOI: 10.4324/9781003279297-5

believer". Religious dogma legitimises the melancholic choice of the depressive patient.

"Mourning and Melancholia" (Freud, 1917) was the great turning point in analytic theorising; it substituted, without excluding it, the paradigm of object relation for that of infantile sexuality; this metapsychological essay had infinite repercussions for the development of analytic theory and practice. The title of this Freudian text is perfectly explicit and deserves to be unfolded: it says that mourning is temporally primary. It is a requirement of reality as imperative as the prohibition of incest, that the loved object, lost, must be abandoned, "disinvested", says Freud; melancholia, on the contrary, is both the refusal of this renunciation and its opposite, since, when the loss of the object proves to threaten the subject's survival, the melancholic process, which is an activity, preserves it, through introjection. As tenacious as this implantation of the beloved object is, thus becoming an internal object, as sophisticated as this operation of introjection is, the conservation of the object is not in any way contradictory with its erasure. In the chapter "The Dependent Relationships of the Ego" of the essay "The Ego and the Id", Freud, while recognising the difficulty of finding the lost and hidden loved object, does not exclude the possibility of it.

The struggle against the obstacle of unconscious guilt is not made easy for the analyst. The analyst can do nothing against it directly and indirectly nothing but slowly uncover its repressed unconscious foundations. There is a particular opportunity to exert influence when this guilt is a borrowed feeling, that is, the result of identification with another person who was once the object of erotic investment. This feeling of guilt is often the unique and hardly recognisable remnant of the abandoned love relationship. Patience, and trust in the analytical process and in the formidable power of the transference to remobilise the most archaic and violently repressed object relations are sure means of thwarting the obstacle that the depressive patient – and his or her apparent psychic desert – puts up against the analytic listening.

On the other hand, "Mourning and Melancholia" initiates an extension of the knowledge of deep psychic layers that makes it go towards the dramatic origins of individual and collective humanity, perhaps towards what Pierre Fédida calls the dehumanisation. One thinks of Georges Bataille at Lascaux who, one of the first to enter this sanctuary, overwhelmed by the strength of the figures represented there, exclaimed, "but these men speak to us, their descendants", and who immediately saw in the cave's parietal engravings the exact passage between animal and man; one might think that melancholia, in any depressive state, would re-actualise the memory of these times. Behind the figure of the dehumanisation we can understand the fear that coloured the first awakening of the mind, that primitive and profound pain that the German calls *Schwermut*, the despair of being still without a god *atheos*.

What makes the unity of depressive states, despite their clinical polymorphism, is not the erasure of all psychic life, but its negation, knowing that negation is an extremely sophisticated operation that engages language in its function of counter-investment of displeasure, of containment of pain and anxiety, an engagement that demobilises in proportion its function of enunciation. A bit like a country at war, which mobilises its peasants and creates famine by turning its countryside into a desert. This operation of language that is negation depends neither on the intention nor on the will of the subject but on a psychic automatism, very deeply inscribed in the very aim of the psychic apparatus, undoubtedly in line with the tendency asserted in "Instincts and their Vicissitudes" to discharge itself from all excitation. The analgesia to which we can reduce the extinction of all psychic life, the loss of the human, deprives the depressive patient of his capacity to experience his feelings and naturally it also deprives him of "the words to say them". Here again, the analyst's response is to tolerate the patient's silence or the hermeticism or apparent emptiness of his or her speech, not as a "refusal" to speak but as a means of experimenting, of getting to know the operations of negation which, within the patient, work to sedate his or her pain and despair, and to restore his or her enthusiasm. It is impossible not to imagine that, in silence, psychic activity does not unfold on a stage other than language, and this other stage is the stage of the image. We note in passing that the analytic process cannot fail to awaken this pain and thereby induces resistance to the analytic work.

The negation of the depressive patient puts him out of all social life: it is the cost of avoiding pain. It will be necessary to examine in detail the multiple facets of this work of negation that, in the cure, the word accomplishes with the operation of silence where it becomes an act, contributing to the desexualisation of the primary oedipal affect. This clarification is the current task of metapsychological research. Let us say that it gives back to language the magical power that the first men discovered in it and that, out of deference, they attributed to their gods. Aeschylus (2014) in *Prometheus in Chains*, to humiliate the rebel for his claim to be equal to the gods, has Hermes say: "The word of Zeus cannot lie: every word that comes out of his mouth is fulfilled". What does this mean if not that in its "accomplishment" through negation, language is no longer enunciation but "act".

References

Aeschylus. (2014). *Théâtre complet*, Paris: GF-Flammarion, p. 125.
Freud, S. (1917). Deuil et mélancolie, *OCF-P*, XIII, Paris: PUF, 1988.

6 The psychoanalysis of a chronically and severely depressed patient

Or "Don't even *think* of coming close!"

Bernard Reith

Severe chronic depression

Mr. B. asked for psychoanalytic treatment for recurrent major depressions that began in adolescence and probably earlier. The more severe episodes were like solitary confinement in a black prison cell. Suicidal thoughts were part of the picture. Between episodes, he never felt fully alive. He had received medication for the worst depressions but, apart from some symptomatic relief, it had not made him feel better. He suffered from chronic anxiety and self-criticism. He knew that he had a role in his depressions through his tendency to sabotage his life, work, and relationships.

He recalled a childhood nightmare in which he was face-to-face with a beast like a wolf with open jaws and sharp teeth and thought that this could be about his father's angry outbursts. In our first interviews Mr. B. came across as proud, even a bit defiant, which could indeed be taken as transference to me as a father. But the gaping jaws featured oral terror. In retrospect the message behind his dignified attitude was: "Don't even *think* of coming close to me – it would be far too painful, frightening and enraging."

Early trauma

Mr. B.'s childhood was characterised by emotional deprivation even if, as he has recently been able to see, his hard-working Latin American parents were also, in their own way, caring and attentive. They had overcome many hardships to build their life, which they protected through rigid normalcy in a secluded nuclear family with their only child. In analysis, Mr. B. came to understand that his father's surveillance and scathing criticism were motivated by anxiety for his future, hoping that study would ensure well-being.

Mr. B.'s mother seemed easily overwhelmed, withdrawing in anxiety or irritation from difficult situations. She had a good job but otherwise restricted her life to watching television and collecting butterflies, which she caught herself, and to which we will come back later. She was often depressed, so post-partum or early motherhood depressions may have played a role. When

DOI: 10.4324/9781003279297-6

Mr. B. asked her whether she had breast-fed him, more than by her negative answer, he was struck by how she gave it, as if it were unimportant.

Mr. B. has memories of being alone while his parents were at work, already before primary school. He managed with heroic daydreams where he was king of the hill, needing no one. Another unconscious defence, however, and which remains one of his main retreats in times of trouble, was to imagine a perfectly ideal, safe place, with a wonderfully sweet, plentiful mother figure, who would gratify any needs or desires before he even had them.

A shy and studious latency was followed by mobbing at school against which he felt defenceless during preadolescence, then a rebellious adolescence. He managed to attain a good level of professional development through courage and reliance on his capacities.

Transference and countertransference dynamics

Although Mr. B. first experienced the couch as a liberation, it soon became clear that anger and resentment were central to his equilibrium, as if these were the only feelings he could afford to have. There were spiteful stories about his childhood and his aging parents. It was difficult for him to stay in touch, but he berated himself for neglecting them.

Resentment infiltrated his work, where Mr. B. would procrastinate and be difficult with his colleagues and superiors, only to be overwhelmed by near-delusional convictions that he would be fired. At times I shared his fears when he really seemed to be endangering his post.

He could not afford to like or love women as persons. His exquisite appreciation of their femininity (the curve of a neck, the fine shape of a hand) aroused dreams of a perfect relationship, but if a real woman loved him, he would panic and find reasons to devalue and hate her.

The analytic relationship could be challenging. Mr. B. could greet me with a resentful glare, miss sessions without warning, make subtle fun of what I said or keep on talking as if I had not spoken. He had several mobile phones with him, which he did not turn off. In one session, he remained silent, answered a call for an animated conversation in a language I didn't understand, then remained silent again until time was up. As much as feeling excluded, my countertransference experience was of falling into a void and disappearing as a person. I took this as reflecting Mr. B.'s experience of not existing for me, as well as his need to fight against me so that I would not exist for him. This fight could be so intense that he was unable to remember what we had talked about from one session to the next, or even from one moment to another in a session.

But he felt guilty about how he treated me. When I interpreted that he thought I was too busy in my mind to be interested in him, or that he felt powerless to build a relationship with me, he would cry softly. Next day, however, this seemed to be forgotten and if I mentioned it, he would change the subject.

Melancholic organisations

These dynamics were not only narcissistic. Mr. B.'s combination of self-destructiveness and guilt were easier to understand as expressing a melancholic organisation.

In Freud's (1917, 1923) model of melancholia, the subject defends against the work of mourning the loss of an ambivalently loved object, or deep disappointment by the object, by identifying with it. He installs the object as part of his personality where he attacks it, thus attacking himself. One source of Mr. B.'s self-criticism was his identification with his father, after his disillusionment with a father he loved and needed but who badly hurt him. The deeper source, as we will see, was a tormented encounter with a primary maternal object.

A closer reading of Freud's model, and of the internal world of severely depressed patients, suggests that things are more complicated. The attacked internal object exerts revenge, becoming an unforgiving superego berating the subject. What we see is not only an internalised object, but an internalised *object relationship* where both subject and object can be attacker and attacked, superego and ego, sadist and victim. My first extension of the model is that melancholia is not so much a structure as a constantly active *dynamic*, a *danse macabre*, expressing a characteristic *pattern* or *quality* of object relationships.

A second and related extension is that this melancholic dance is often more *enacted* than represented. It is active in our patients' inner world but also in their everyday lives, as when Mr. B. was compelled to damage his life and his reputation. I soon realised how this dance could infect the analytic relationship, when well-intended interpretations came out as slightly sharp, judgmental, or reproachful.

Mr. B.'s phobia of butterflies illustrated such melancholic object relations. He was afraid they might touch him and believed he could break their wings if he brushed them away. As a child, he had watched his mother pin them to a board and inject them with formaldehyde to kill and embalm them. He was afraid that I would pin him to the couch with devastating pronouncements about his mind, while I worried that I could push him to suicide with a wrong interpretation. In turn, he pinned me to my analyst's chair when he behaved as if I did not exist. The elegant female hands he loved were the hands his mother used to kill, but he would be the one who nailed women sexually in his imagination, only to leave them for dead when they loved him. The needle was a paradoxical image of his need for contact with an unreachable and infanticidal primary object. Broken wings and death expressed fears of breakdown and annihilation.

Breakdown

This brings us to my third extension of the model. It is difficult to understand why one would be so invested in maintaining violent internal dynamics unless they are a psychic retreat (Steiner 1993) against some greater danger. For

Freud it was the unbearable pain of mourning. Like others, I suggest that the danger is breakdown (Press 2019; Winnicott 1974). Breakdown can follow loss, but also disturbances of the *encounter* with the object. The melancholic subject hangs on to destructive internal objects not only because presence is better than absence; he idealises their destructiveness to build a dam against breakdown, and their omnipotence as a bastion against vulnerability.

We were between Charybdis and Scylla. Mr. B.'s melancholic defences, aroused by the analysis and manifested through lateral transferences, threatened his everyday life, so it was necessary to interpret them. And yet, doing so exposed him to the internal traumatic situation he was struggling to avoid.

The threat of breakdown first came out as un-representable terror. At times near the end of the first year of analysis Mr. B. literally stank of fear. It wasn't just that he could be too depressed to shower or launder his clothes. This was a different smell, more like that of a terrified prey hoping to disgust a predator.

Breakdown came in the second year, as the deepest and longest depressive phase of the analysis, after a failed love relationship led him to realise how devastating his defences could be. Like the anxiety, this was a profoundly physical state. To explain how he felt when alone in bed at night, he said that "even the air I breathe is filled with pain". There was a component of regression in the service of the analysis, allowing him to share his deep distress with me, but the situation was dangerous. Despite his reassurances, I was sure that he was suicidal. He only confirmed years later that he had in fact all along kept the means in his bedside drawer to die efficiently, painlessly, and in silence. Mr. B. accepted to consult a psychiatrist for medication, and I was grateful that I had set this condition as part of our agreement in case depression endangered his life or his ability to work with me. He was able to stop medication after two years and since then has no longer needed this colleague.

Embodied phenomena

We had no choice but to hold on. Mr. B.'s breakdown took us down to the most basic level of psychic functioning, where the body is the locus of experience and where object relationships are first experienced and integrated.

Much of this primordial experience is registered as unconscious ways of being (Matte-Blanco 1988), which are not represented in the usual sense, but which the analyst can learn to capture in his own inner experience to let their meaning emerge and find ways to symbolise them which the patient may be able to use. This level has been explored from many perspectives (Bion 1962, 1967; Castoriadis-Aulagnier 1975; Isaacs 1948; Leuzinger-Bohleber 2019; Ogden 1989; Roussillon 1999; Tustin 1992). As background to this symbolising function, psychoanalytic work may also involve more pre-reflective work where the analyst's resonance with, but toleration of, archaic defences help him to respond flexibly and allow new possibilities to emerge.

Such work takes time. A session from the fourth year of analysis, for example, began with a dog he saw playing joyfully with its mistress in a park. This led to a television program about coyotes with impressive jaws, a new secretary at work whom he found attractive but who seemed vulnerable, and healthy-looking Nordic blondes whose origins he linked to what he supposed about mine. Then came a final and frightening shift to a TV report about a farmer who beat calves to death to prove his strength. There was a photo of him carrying a dead calf on his shoulders. That was criminal, Mr. B. said: they should put him in prison.

Together we could trace the movement from joyful and energetic contact to his fear of being voracious and destructive, and therefore needing me to be reassuringly strong. But the last scene was a plunge into a zone where contact could only be cruel and shattering.

Two sessions in the sixth year of analysis

The sessions I will report in detail are from a time when Mr. B.'s life was globally improving, but he was more depressed again, albeit not as severely as in the past.

At the beginning of the Monday session, he spoke slowly and hesitantly, in a distant and hollow tone, affecting me with mixed feelings of impatience, exclusion, and unreality.

Mr. B.: "I'm thinking that I can't figure out what my state of mind is, and I'm hoping you will be able to tell me. [Silence.] I've been wanting to call my mother lately, but I haven't called her all weekend."

He described important professional projects that he should attend to, and which could endanger his post and hence the analysis if he delayed too much. He talked about this with discouragement and despair. He had spent the entire weekend watching television series, seeing this as his attempt to connect with his emotions.

I said: "It is difficult for you to connect with me after the weekend. You need us to work together to figure out what state of mind you are in, but you are not sure you can trust that, so you think you have to do it alone, by watching television. You are afraid that because of your difficulty contacting me, the analysis will come to an end."

After a silence, M. B. said: "I never thought that finding out what state of mind I'm in could be something we could do together. I always thought I had to do it alone. [Silence.] It's true what you say about my difficulty connecting with you. I can recognise that feeling with my mother. That's why I don't call her." [Silence.]

Something about his tone led me to say: "You feel you can't trust connecting with me, because you don't know whether it will be helpful or painful."

Mr. B.'s reaction was spectacular. His whole body became tense and shook, as if he were sobbing, which was not the case so far as I could tell. It was a long spasm which increased in frequency before subsiding. After a while he balled his fists. He hit them together a few times; then, he hit the left side of his chest with his right fist several times over. Afterwards he lay more calmly, remaining silent.

My impression was that he was expressing anger, anxiety and pain, in a confused mixture. I was struck by what looked like beating his heart and silently copied his gesture behind the couch to understand it. Although I don't usually interpret behaviour, after a while I decided this was too important to let it pass unmentioned.

ME: "Did you want to tell me something by beating your heart?"
MR. B.: "What do you mean?"
ME: "You beat your chest, near your heart, with your fist."
MR. B.: "I wasn't aware I did that." [Silence.]
ME: "I believe you became tense, because there was something wrong in what I said about wanting to connect with me and not knowing whether it would turn out well or not. I think what is closer to how you feel is that in all cases you expect it to be painful."

After another silence, Mr. B. said: "Yes, I can recognise that feeling. It is how I feel about calling my mother. I always expect it to be disappointing. That's what my thoughts are about when I think about calling her."

Letting my own body speak up through my mouth, I said: "Yes, and it is more than your thoughts, it is also physical. Just now, when we were talking about making contact, you became very tense. It was as if instead of feeling your heart beat because you want contact, or having it broken if that doesn't work, you feel it's better to beat your heart yourself. It's safer that way."

Mr. B. seemed moved but remained silent. His mobile phone rang, he turned it off, and remained silent again. As we were nearing the end of the hour, he put his wristwatch back on, his sign that he knows it will soon be time. Then he had another gesture which was new to me: he interlocked his fingers tightly as in prayer, then pulled on his hands as if to make sure that they would hold together.

I thought about leaving well enough alone, but this new gesture also seemed important. I said: "You are aware we're near the end of the hour and you are holding your hands as if to hold yourself together until tomorrow. And maybe you are also holding on to me."

Mr. B. responded with yet another gesture: he cupped one hand in the other and stroked it. Then he interlocked his fingers again.

He looked moved when we said goodbye.

Next day

Next day, Mr. B. seemed livelier. He described how he had set the alarm clock at five a.m. that morning to make headway on a business plan that was worrying him, although morning is the time of day when he is least efficient. He fell asleep again after five minutes, which he described as another failure. Then, he dreamt that he was talking with someone and solving problems. "But now", he said, "I still have to do that project."

While wondering privately about the ambivalent transference meaning of the dream, I asked him whether it wasn't a bit cruel to force himself to work so early in the morning, if he knew it wasn't the best time for him.

Mr. B. rationalised a bit but then said: "But you are right, it is cruel. I'm often cruel with myself. [Long silence.] I was silent because I was thinking about Martin Scorsese's film *Raging Bull* with Robert de Niro. It's about a boxer who seemed to get more satisfaction from his ability to stand getting beaten up, than beating his adversaries. He has this incredible capacity to take punches without falling. It's like he's proud of that." [Silence.]

ME: "You can feel like him?"

MR. B.: "Yes, in a way. It's based on the life of Jake La Motta. He was a man with problems, with the Mafia and alcohol. There's a scene in prison where he beats his fists against the wall, hurting himself, so in a way he is beating himself. He scolds himself while he does that, calling himself stupid."

ME: "That could remind us of my impression yesterday that you were beating yourself on the heart."

MR. B.: "Well, I wouldn't be so stupid as to punch a wall, I wouldn't want to damage my hands. But sometimes when I look in the mirror, I slap myself in the face and tell myself I'm stupid. It hurts, but it doesn't do physical damage."

ME: "On a day like yesterday when you feel you can't reach me, you feel like I'm a concrete prison wall and you can't get through to me even by punching. You feel it's stupid even to try because it will only make you hurt more, so you prefer to hit yourself."

After a silence, Mr. B. said: "I don't know what to make of that comment", but he sounded much moved.

ME: "You feel my comment is stupid, but you are also moved, and maybe you feel stupid about feeling moved. When you want to be with me, you can feel stupid to want that because you are convinced it will only bring pain. Maybe when you want to call your mother, and are afraid it will go wrong, you feel stupid about wanting to call her."

Mr. B. balled his right hand into a fist, then cupped it in his left hand and stroked it, then stroked both hands. He locked his fingers together for a moment and wiped away a tear. After a while, he said: "Before, those scenes where he lets himself get bashed, I found them exciting. Now, I only find them sad." [Long silence.] "You know, I have this golden retriever soft toy from when I was a kid. Well, this morning I put it to bed, its head on the pillow, and tucked its body under the blanket. I was thinking just now, to take care of my soft toy like that, but to bash myself, well, *that is* stupid."

Later developments

Three years later, I still think of these sessions as a turning point. The analytic relationship became more alive. Mr. B.'s body spoke more, adding depth to our work. We also came to understand the discharge function of his previous uses of his body to evacuate all needs and desires and reach a state of "flatness" as he described it. He needed to do so because, when he needed relationships, his overpowering fear was of getting lost in some vast empty space where nothing made sense.

We have seen how Mr. B. reacts not only to my absences and failures, but also to my *presence*, which arouses fears of distress and breakdown as much as my mistakes or the gaps between hours. To my dismay I sometimes enacted fears about closeness, prematurely ending a session when emotional contact was deepening, or when we could finally laugh together. He understood what was happening and this was another major turning point.

Over the past two years Mr. B. has been able to maintain, with great apprehension and ambivalence, a difficult but affectionate love relationship. Once, describing his tormented feelings about her, he said that he wanted to "tear [his] heart out of [his] chest".

Primary identification

The soft toy that Mr. B. tucks in bed, the playful dog, the coyotes, the dead calf, and embalmed butterflies all seem to represent aspects of the same profoundly disturbed infantile experience. Hitting a prison wall, being beaten to death, or injected and embalmed, point to states of agony and annihilation. The spasms may repeat archaic physical reactions to distress.

My fourth extension of our model of melancholia concerns the identifications that are involved. Freud's model describes a *secondary* identification with an object which, although narcissistic, has been at least partially constituted as distinct from the self before its reincorporation. Severe melancholic states may be better understood if we see the secondary identifications as taking root in more *primary* identifications. Rather than phantasies about as yet poorly differentiated objects, what matters most in primary identification is the *sensual state* of the relationship. The mother's reverie and holding and the infant's responses have a reciprocal dynamic where self and object, passive and active experience, are consubstantial and indistinguishable, forming the groundwork for all subsequent self- and object-representations. If something goes wrong at this level, this wrongness *becomes part of the self.* A repetitively painful state of primary relationships may become a template for the developing ego and paradoxically a secure bedrock to which to regress in times of trouble.

This view has helped me to understand Mr. B.'s defences and his difficulty in relinquishing them.

References

Bion, W. R. (1962). *Learning from experience.* London: Karnac.
Bion, W. R. (1967). *Second thoughts.* London: Karnac.
Castoriadis-Aulagnier, P. (1975). *La violence de l'interprétation: Du Pictogramme à l'énoncé.* Paris: P.U.F.
Freud, S. (1917 [1915]). Mourning and melancholia. *S.E.* 14: 243–258.
Freud, S. (1923). The ego and the id. *S.E.* 19: 1–66.
Isaacs, S. (1948) The nature and function of phantasy. *International Journal of Psychoanalysis*, 29, 73–97.
Leuzinger-Bohleber, M. (2019). *Finding the body in the mind: Embodied memories, trauma, and depression.* London and New York: Routledge.
Matte-Blanco, I. (1988). *Thinking, feeling and being.* London: Routledge.
Ogden, T. H. (1989). *The primitive edge of experience.* Northvale, NJ: Aronson.
Press, J. (2019). Au-delà de la mélancolie. Mélancolie et crainte de l'effondrement. *Revue française de psychanalyse*, 83, 527–540.
Roussillon, R. (1999). *Agonie, clivage et symbolisation.* Paris: P.U.F.
Steiner, J. (1993). *Psychic retreats: Pathological organisations of the personality in psychotic, neurotic and borderline patients.* London: Routledge.
Tustin, F. (1992) *Autistic states in children.* London: Routledge.
Winnicott, D. W. (1974). Fear of breakdown. *International Review of Psychoanalysis*, 1, 103–107.

7 "Switching the light off to cast the shadow away"

Jean-François Simoneau

As I was preparing my comments of Anne Brun's Sandler lecture, I had shared with her my feelings of the Uncanny as Freud's new 1919 translation, *Das Unheimliche*, would have it. The excerpts chosen were intended to echo her lecture on the disembodiment of melancholic incorporations. I had received her text after having chosen my sequences of analysis and at the same time her text appeared familiar to me, as if it had come out of my clinical work, or rather, it was my clinical work that seemed to come out of her text. It was as if the word of her text conditioned the thing (*das Ding*) of my clinical work! At the same time, I was seized by a gap, a difference that at first appeared irreconcilable before disappearing into the familiar. Perhaps this is what Freud's Uncanny is all about, a play of light and shadow.

Through this piece of analysis presented at the time, I wanted to figure out the incorporative identifications of my patient and the whole work of the treatment consisting, in the first instance, in identifying them and then freeing him from them. I had the melancholic incorporations, but what troubled me was that his superego had remained quite silent for a long time while melancholy was lurking. Indeed, no devastating self-reproaches and loud self-accusations – no, I had to catch an almost inaudible rustle, a "never again", before I heard the sound of a broken instrument, a broken psychic apparatus under the pressure of despair and rage. It is only once the light had been shed on the incorporates and on the reduction of investments that the shadows began to move again, that the objects began to dance, first a macabre dance and then a passionate dance on the floor of transference – a dance whose movements were first felt on the counter-transferential stage.

It was only at this point that I was able to grasp, with my patient, that the breakdown had already taken place and that what was being heard was the echo of a drama that never ceased to repeat itself, that of an immeasurable gap between the shadow and its object, rendering all address lost. It took the transference to cover the object with its shadow, leading to a necessary agony, an obligatory passage to retie the threads of a story and allow the traces of an object to be "found". Or, as Anne Brun says, to bring out a "theatre of shadows" where it is a question of staging the play of shadows and lights, and the disappointments experienced in the encounter(s) with the object.

DOI: 10.4324/9781003279297-7

Jaime was a young man of barely 25 years old when I met him for the first time, a little less than two years ago. He is of Spanish origin and his family divides its life between Switzerland and Andalusia, where Jaime practices his art, the flamenco guitar. He is the eldest of four children. If the link is distant but preserved with his older sister, the relationship with his twin younger brothers is "practically non-existent because they are too different", he will say. His mother also plays the guitar, but Jaime is keen to point out that "even though she is an excellent player, I didn't learn anything from her … It's almost a coincidence that we play the same instrument … I was a complete self-taught until I was 18". Jaime's career unfolds in Andalusia, between Cadiz, Seville and Cordoba. His father is an orthopedic surgeon, sharing his activity between Spain and Switzerland. Jaime contacted me several months after getting my name from his father, who had asked a colleague for addresses for his son, who, according to his father's words to the colleague, "since he came home, has been a real bully with us, especially with his mother". The first time I met Jaime, I was struck by his slim body, without being skinny, slender, without being tall. A body full of nuances but with a very particular posture, it is a little curved in front. Once seated in front of me, I would say to myself that his body envelops his instrument, which creates a music that envelops him in turn, producing a strange image of a Moebius strip where inside and outside, backwards and forwards merge. Jaime doesn't come to tell his story, he's not interested, at least not at first, he comes to live it because, he says, "For almost a year, I've been a shadow of my former self, I don't live anymore … to survive is already too much to say". He quickly shows me by his silences, by his elusive look and his stiffening body that my questions or my looks aimed at getting him going again are putting him under strain. He comes to hear himself, he who "doesn't have the impression of having been heard". It is he who will give the tempo, the rhythm, often jerky, of the words, of the sentences before making an associative thread. He weaves this thread for himself first, as if he were stretching a string on his guitar before making it vibrate and then, only after an often long time, tuning it and an even longer time to make a note of it. Unfolding Jaime's story does not take into account these syncopated elements that I have just mentioned, because in order to tell the story, it is necessary to connect, put together, oppose, clarify, replace or substitute. In short, one must translate primary to secondary thinking. The patient is certainly capable of this. He was, no doubt, from the beginning, but the ordeal of telling another what was taking shape inside him made him suffer because, he would tell me, "When I speak to you, it is torn out of me and it comes out any way … in any case, not the way I hear it in my head". It seems to me that the encounter between psychic reality and historical/material reality suffered, in Jaime, a great porosity. The work of the preconscious seems, at times, to impede the narrative.

The following session, which I consider to be the pivotal one of the analysis, took place eight months ago, about a year after the beginning of the analysis:

Two terrible things happened to me between yesterday and today. First of all, I don't understand what happened to me last night ... I am feverish ... I dreamt of my ex-girlfriend, whereas at the last session I told you that she was, at least that's what I wished you had told me, that she was petrified inside me ... I was no longer in pain ... She was there, inside me. I was going around her but I no longer felt that terrible pain that has been with me since she told me that between us it was impossible ....

I struggled to recognize my patient, this young man, usually restrained, even a little frozen, inhabited by a quest for the right word, while there, sitting on the couch, his head in his hands, he was trembling. I remembered the previous day's session when he had told me coldly that he had petrified his former girlfriend. "Devitalized, turned to stone, inanimate, petrified. Yes, petrified is the right word," he had said, as if relieved.

I then had associations which appeared to me as revealing his agonistic experiences during the almost two years since their separation. First, I had the image of Courbet's painting "Lot and his daughters". Lot's wife had been transformed into a pillar of salt by defying the divine prohibition to turn back on Sodom. I then thought of the petrification of those who, full of curiosity and fear, look at the Medusa for the first and last time ... Another association appeared to me in the form of a railroad convoy transporting vitrified radioactive waste that is being buried ... in the vague hope that the radiation will not return. I was surprised to see myself summoned in this way by the sexual, the traumatic and the overflow or the fear of collapse. I was petrified by the petrification claimed by my patient.

Let us return to this first part of the session, marked by the recounting of the dream. After a few seconds, he continues:

I was in a house in Italy, looking suspiciously like the one we stayed in, with my family last summer. I found my girlfriend in a huge hall. I realize that it is not the house from last year because the one in the dream is much bigger, it is rather the one where I went to give a concert some time before the pandemic in Cadiz ... My girlfriend tells me, very angry, that she is going to leave, that I should not keep her ... I accompany her to the car. I carry her red suitcase and she continues to tell me that this is not possible in a very harsh tone that does not sound like her. She's out of her mind and she's never been like this. I open the trunk of the car and put her red suitcase in the trunk. She is more and more angry and she tries to slap me ... And there, it's incredible, it's me who gives her a slap so strong that she falls forward and topples into the trunk. I close the trunk and leave with the car ... I woke up sweating. I would never have hit her. How is it possible to dream such things ... I never thought about it that way. It was impossible between us, such violence.

After a long silence, I say again "Unthinkable, impossible, it's very different". As if absent, he associates:

When my girlfriend told me that it was impossible between us, that she couldn't leave her husband, that it would hurt him too much, that it would be a change that seemed impossible to accept. For me, this "impossible" was unthinkable. In fact, I didn't understand it right away. It was because I insisted that this situation had lasted long enough and that a new separation, between two series of shows, was too difficult... That's when she told me that it was impossible ... So why, why did she get me on the stage and put up with my harsh words in the first place because I didn't want to be approached. I hadn't asked for anything. She accepted a lot from me before finally we could live our story ... But all this I have already told you. I shouldn't think about it anymore, I'm suffering unnecessarily. Petrifying her, and all that we have been through, is the right solution ... Never again, never again will I let myself be taken....

In the silence that follows, I wonder about what is petrified, the dancing girlfriend, the object of desire or desire itself, the "*Sehnsucht*", the movement, the quest that goes towards the object that never ceases to escape the grasp. We will come back to this.

After a moment of silence, when he is as if petrified on the couch, I say to him: "That red suitcase, something loaded into a trunk". By saying this, I seem to be bringing my patient out of a certain torpor or reverie. "I don't like to think this but red is the color of anger, we say 'red with anger' don't we ... Never, there was a bit of anger between us ...". "Yes, to the unthinkable impossible," I added. "In the dream, she is the one who is angry, who is very hard on me. It's her suitcase...". I intervene, nearly interrupting him: "And it's you who's locking her up". This untimely intervention comes to me as if it were out of character, it confuses me. After some hesitation, he continued:

You're right, I'm angry, I'm mad at her for letting me in and then kicking me out, telling me "It's not possible between us" ... But to lock her up is to take her with me, everywhere, all the time. It's been almost two years since it ended ... I can't go on like this, she's always there, I'm exhausted ... I never said it but it has to stop ... Never, I could have shown or said it before. I never show or say anything, often I don't feel anything and when I do feel, it's terrible, it's beyond me.

There is a lot to say about this very condensed dream, which takes up whole sections of my patient's history and which reveals, for the first time, in a way that is audible to him, it seems to me, what René Roussillon (1998) calls energetic neutralization. Indeed, the petrification attempted by my patient would be one of the modes of figuration of a defensive organization trying to prevent the return of states of lack that could have degenerated into states of distress, or even into primitive agonies. This threat to the ego requires the restriction of investments and relationships in order to protect oneself from the return of these agonies, caused by the effects of loss or divergence inherent in all relationships. This "never again" condenses, as we will see later, a past and a future, an overload before and a cut-off after.

It is the second event announced by my patient at the beginning of the session that will put us on the track of the traces that petrification tries to neutralize. The tears barely dry, he stiffens, stops breathing. His limbs tighten and I see his fists clench and his knuckles turn white from the strain. In a faint voice, he says, "The height of disaster happened to me this afternoon". He had been rehearsing for several hours for a show with a dancer that will be broadcasted, because of the pandemic, and he decided to put his instrument down in the same place, with the same rotational movement that he has done, he tells me, "thousands of times" over the years ... "And then, my instrument hits something and cracks". He seems to be reliving the scene as he swings his head around.

> I didn't dare to move. Then I turned my head and saw that an iron spike had pierced the chamber of my instrument. A decorative spike from a coffee table that had never been there before. My immediate thought was: this is my mother. My mother did that. I don't have to ask her, I'm sure.

His conviction that his mother did this is unquestionable. It signs a confession. His mother can enter his home, inside him. The stone becomes flint and begins to speak by cutting the heart of its instrument. "I'm sure my instrument will lose its voice after a blow like that. It is lost. I went to my luthier here, he told me, that after the repair, we won't hear anything". But my patient knows that it will never be the same again. For him, the voice of his instrument is lost, "forever". I hesitate between "being" next to him and echoing what is happening in order to bear, together, this nameless distress or interpret this castration. The silence is prolonged and I feel agitation rising within me. I do not exclude that this agitation is the one that the patient cannot allow himself to live. I decide to propose a bridge, a sketch of a link that passes through the act and I say: "A girlfriend who gets spiked and slapped; a mother who spikes and goes through a safe!" After a brief silence and a deep breath, the patient ends the session by murmuring, as if to himself, "I always knew it but I didn't want to see it, I let this woman into my fortress. I should never have let her in. She was already in ...". A little louder, the condemnation falls: "If it loses its voice, I kill her". He gets up and, forgetting about Covid, shakes my hand warmly.

This session, a turning point if ever there was one, opened up all sorts of questions about the voice and the path to take ... Which voice is it? The voice of the instrument, of the former girlfriend, of the mother? And which instrument is he talking about? The present one? All the others that were martyred to fit the shape of his body? Or on another level, is there a difference between the music, the instrument and him? To ask these questions is to solve the enigma of a murder. And again, what murder is it? Recalling what Freud wrote in 1912 that "No one can be killed in absentia or in effigy". And if there was a murder, was it in self-defense? The following sessions will take up, in a different way, the beginnings of the story and what will happen in the future. Let us remember that this session took place about a year after the beginning of the treatment. While I am still shaken by the last session, my patient arrives at the next one and says he is "reassured".

> I don't know what happened, but since the last session I feel better ... My instrument will be ready next week ... the luthier is reassuring ... we'll see .... My mother confirmed what I knew, she set the table for me to put my cup of tea down as I was said to be marking the floor ... I didn't say anything but I thought she had what she wanted ....

"What did she want? To pierce your mystery ..." I said to him, surprising myself by such suggestive audacity. In fact, by saying this, I was giving substance to an oedipal mother, which did not yet appear to me at that time, or to an intrusive mother, an echo of my patient's defense. I attributed my precipitation of the moment on the effect of fright of the petrification of the previous session. This is the premise of my failure to come. I can now return to the sessions following the pivotal session of the dream and the two condemnations, the petrification and the threat of murder. During these sessions, Jaime and I will be able to excavate the conditions of the encounter of his first love, of this first woman, and this from a failure on my part. In fact, as I pointed out, I had remained "petrified" by my patient's desired petrification of his former girlfriend and by the announcement of the death sentence if he lost his voice? In retrospect, I realize that I took these two condemnations literally and they stayed with me during the following sessions, as a potential threat of acting out. It was in this context, as I mentioned, that during the next session of the dream and the peak in the instrument, I found myself interpreting an oedipal and/or intrusive mother. The implacable logic behind this signifying sequence fuels my patient's "never again". "Never again will I invest myself. Never again will I let anyone into my world", is the refrain that Jaime would repeat over the few months that followed.

As I watch the analysis get bogged down in "never again", Jaime, who has resumed traveling to Andalusia for a series of shows, asks for a session to be changed to allow him to travel to Cadiz. The window on the pandemic helps me to accept this departure from the setting. However, the sanitary conditions in Spain worsened and the concert was cancelled. Jaime tells me this, and asks me to restore the canceled session. I agree but do not enter the information in my diary. On the date of the session, I find Jaime and another patient in the waiting room. I realize my mistake. Jaime withdraws without saying a word and returns two days later for the rescheduled session. He settles in and remains silent for what seems like a longer time than usual. I brace myself for an angry salvo over my failure and he begins:

> I was early today and I went to the park next door. There was a couple kissing. It was awkward. It was like I wasn't there. I turned my head away and heard them arguing. When I turned around, she was gone and the young man smiled at me and continued to eat his sandwich.

After a silence, I resume: "The last time, you went away and left this patient and me alone, like a boy who feels like he is too much ... although it was your place, your time."

> I don't know what you're talking about ... Ah, if it's about the last session, it was me who asked you to change. So, it was my fault in the first place ... Anyway, it's all in the past now. It's all closing up again, in Spain, it's going to lock up again. It's over. It will never be like it was before.

His tone is unambiguous. I hesitate between underlining the closing movement of "never again" which seems to seal the first manifestation of negative transference and open up the primitive scene, represented by the deflection of his gaze in the park or his muffled departure when I took the other patient. Aware that the two dimensions are linked by despair, I attempt an interpretative thread. "This couple, it's the one of your parents who kissed and argued, it's also the one you formed with your girlfriend. Spikes and kisses alternate and you remain alone in your fortress of 'never again', as here ..." I don't have time to add the sequel that builds in me around the violence he's inflicting on himself before he interrupts me.

> I already told you that my parents have nothing to do with this. They fought a lot, it's true, my father almost died because my mother was so unbearable, but my friend has nothing to do with my parents, and even less with my mother. Nothing, I tell you, nothing to do with her. I don't even know why I'm so upset about what you're saying ... I shouldn't feel anything because there's nothing ...

He sits down on the edge of the couch, as if ready to leave ... He lies down again, sits up, looks as if he wants to get up and then lies down again ... "You've already tried to shut down that impotent rage and we know that's the best way to keep it inside you when you wish it would go away ... To silence that voice, you have to let it speak ..." In this movement back and forth on the couch, I see my patient again when he tells me about the dream in which he had slapped his former girlfriend. I see him again with his head in his hands, telling me for the first time that he could not take it anymore. It is this impotent rage that appears to me as the voice. The voice of the instrument, of the music and of the mother. A voice that kills him and protects him at the same time. To lose it, you have to make it your own. The paradox of loss.

> You don't understand anything, my former girlfriend has let me down, like I was nothing to her. I won't be caught out again. That's what I told myself the other day when I walked out of the office when you took the other patient. I wanted to believe that I was important to you and that didn't stop you from acting as if nothing happened. As you can see, my

parents have nothing to do with this, they are always there even if they don't know what to do with me ...

While I hesitate to explore the powerlessness of the parents, like my own, Jaime evokes what seems to be a *"fueros"*, those early memory traces, which seem to me to point more to a state of affect than to a real memory. "I'm used to seeing my parents' dismay at me, especially when I'd get all worked up because I wanted to go fishing and they didn't have time to go with me, or when I'd bite my guitar because it didn't sound the way I wanted..." And suddenly he's banging his head on the couch and banging his closed fists on it.

I have an image that comes back to me, it came back to me before, a long time ago, but why now. I'm in my bed with bars and I can hardly stand on my legs, I'm screaming, I'm between sleep and wakefulness, my parents are there, they don't dare approach me, they tell me to wake up or go back to bed ... These were my night terrors, for several years, between 2 and 7 years old, I had this, several times. I had the sensation of diluting myself in space ... Never, I could tell them but that was it, I was afraid of getting lost in space...

To lose oneself in space, to lose oneself in the other ... Perhaps this is the "never again" that we talk about so much. How to be in connection with the other, to need it, without fearing to get lost in it, to get caught in it, forever. The transference opened a breach in the fortress and since then the analytical work has been able to take off again on a ridge path, bordered on one side by important rationalizations, allowing the patient an illusion of control by his intelligence, and on the other, fears of overflowing if he lets himself go in the relationship.

References

Freud, S. (1912). The dynamics of transference. *S.E.* 12: 99–108.
Roussillon, R. (1998). *Agonie, clivage et symbolisation* (Chapter 1, pp. 7–39). Paris: PUF.

8   Getting out of the shadow of the object

Anne Brun

Let us listen to a poet, Henri Michaux, who describes better than any psychiatric book the subjective experience of patients suffering from chronic depression in a poem entitled *La Ralentie (the Slowed down)*:

"One is the Slowed down [...] Cannot, does not have any more part in anything [...] something constrains somebody". "One has its hollow elsewhere" "One has given up its place to the shade..." "One collects its disappeared, come, come." "One does not dream any more. One is dreamed. Silence". "I am the shadow of a shadow which is stuck ..." (1963, 573–580).

I propose to enter into what Henri Michaux calls "the space of shadows" (1963, 515–527), rather than reducing chronic depression to a recognizable mental disorder, rather than inventorying its forms, by operating a fine psychiatric semiology. My aim is to identify a common problem in all chronic depression, beyond the singularity of the subjects, their pathologies and their history. The central axis of this communication is inspired by Freud who describes melancholia by this famous metaphor: "The shadow of the object fell upon the ego" (1917, p. 270).

Without reducing chronic depression to the entity of melancholia, we will see melancholic processes at work, or rather melancholic incorporations in different forms of chronic depression that cover different clinical configurations. Freud had already pointed out that, even in descriptive psychiatry, the concept of melancholia is defined in different manners, and that it "occurs in diverse clinical forms which it is not certain that they can be brought together in a unity" (Ibid., p. 263).

I will thus deploy the somewhat enigmatic question of the shadow of the object that falls on the ego, following contemporary analytic works, notably the work by D.W. Winnicott, D. Anzieu, P. Aulagnier and R. Roussillon: my first thread will consist of identifying from my clinical work the main figures of the shadow of the object that falls upon the ego and of evoking some directions of the analytic technique to free oneself, patient as well as analyst, from this shadow of the object that also falls on the analytic treatment. The psychotherapeutic work consists thus, according to a formulation of Roussillon (2019), in "disincarcerating", in "disincorporating" the shadow of the object, by bringing back on scene the conditions of historical meeting of the infant with his objects. We will see that the analytic work consists precisely in

DOI: 10.4324/9781003279297-8

illuminating the zones of indifferentiation with the object, which makes it possible to free the subject vampirized by the shadow of its objects.

My second thread, woven with the first, will be based on the hypothesis that, in order to be able to treat chronic depression, the work of psycho-analytic therapy goes through a kind of shadow theater, which allows the shadow or shadows with which the patient is identified to be brought to light, to be contemplated on an external screen, to be put on stage and into a story. To use the title of a book by Joyce McDougall (1982), the "Theaters of the Mind" become a shadow theater so that the subject suffering from chronic depression can emerge in his or her singularity and deploy his or her aborted potentialities, swallowed up by the shadow.

Shadow of the object and melancholic process: Freud

In his famous article "Mourning and Melancholia" (1915–1917), written in the wake of the introduction of narcissism (1914), Freud associates the deeply painful depression that characterizes melancholia with a

> diminution of the sense of self-worth that manifests itself in self-reproaches. An essential point is the hatred of the melancholic for himself: these self-reproaches are reproaches against an object of love, which are reversed from this one on the proper ego.
>
> (p. 269)

This hatred of the object thus turns against the ego which will identify itself with the abandoned object. Freud formulates this identification of the ego with the abandoned object in a grasping way: "The shadow of the object fell upon the ego" (p. 270). The object is then internalized, incorporated in what Freud designates as a narcissistic identification: one could add that this narcissistic identification is fundamentally an incorporative identification. In this process, the disappointment in relation to the idealized object plays an essential role: the ego, disappointed by the object, identifies then with this object, incorporated in him and abandoned outside.

But Freud does not wonder about the role of the object nor about the relational modalities of the object with the subject that could lead the shadow of this object to fall on the ego. In other words, why does the object turn out to be disappointing? The answer to this question presumes to question the historical reality of the first link with the object and not just the psychological mechanisms at work in the melancholic subject. The shadow of the object will not fall in the same way, according to the characteristics of this object.

Moreover, Freud evokes a loss of the object of love in the melancholic patient, but it is an enigmatic loss, "hidden from consciousness", he writes. In fact, the problematic of the lost object proposed by Freud in this text concerns especially mourning and not melancholia. In melancholia, it is the disappointment which causes the incorporation of the object. Roussillon (2009,

2019) emphasizes that this disappointment does not concern the absence of the object but its mode of presence: the disappointing object, evoked by Freud, is thus differentiated from an absent object.

Freud notes the way in which the melancholic patient is split into one part of the ego that opposes the other and he notes that it is the "moral aversion of the patient towards his own ego that is in the foreground" (p. 268). In 1921, in "Group Psychology and the Analysis of the Ego", Freud returns to his proposal of "Mourning and Melancholia", and evokes the hatred of the object for the subject that is unleashed against the subject, precisely when the object is incorporated. Freud will take up this question in "The Ego and the Id" (1923), by showing that the feeling of intense guilt in melancholia refers to the violent criticism of the superego that is unleashed against the ego: the ego then feels hated and persecuted by the superego. Freud writes that "a pure culture of death drive reigns now in the superego" (1923, p. 268), which can then lead the ego to destruction and death. In other words, the parent internalized in the superego knows the subject's hidden desires and treats them as acts, which blocks any way out since the desires can no longer even be realized in representation. Melancholia results from this deadlock because representation is treated as an act. It is thus the superego that carries the cruelty and the invisible destructive shadow of the object.

To approach the enigma of the shadow that falls on the ego, I will start from my clinical practice with melancholic incorporates. This clinical work necessarily raises issues of narcissism and identity, as we have just seen.

Figure of the shadow of the object in chronic depression

Figure of the shadow of a persecuting object: I am the Evil

A persecuting shadow

A patient of mine, a medical doctor in her thirties, asks for analytical work because, while everything is going well professionally and in her relationship which has lasted for several years, she regularly sinks into depression where she sees everything in black. She describes her relationship with her partner as idyllic, fusional; the only problem is that he works too much, he loves his job and often stays there very late, he wants to achieve a brilliant career. She recalls violent scenes in her early childhood, with a separation of her parents. It was her mother who had left her father for her stepfather. Her father had to leave the marital home, he never recovered from this rupture and lives alone. Mrs. A. has always hated her stepfather, a man described as violent, angry, very severe with her and disqualifying. As a child, she was often alone, waiting for her mother who worked very late. She says she took refuge in school work.

In the first year of analysis, she vehemently reproaches her boyfriend for not taking care of her: he suddenly wants to marry her and have a child. But he was always very unavailable and she finally left him some time later, telling him that she needed a break to think. Shortly after, she discovers that he had started a relationship with another woman. Sessions of real tsunami of passion, with crying, screaming, crazy suffering, with a lot of rage, powerlessness and extreme distress follow.... She feels denied, erased in one stroke, replaced in an interchangeable way. She tries to see him again but comes up against "a wall of ice".

She continues to say that she loves her ex-boyfriend; she vehemently accuses herself of having lost this man she loved, and this is irremediable, which is too much pain for her. She can say at this time that the analysis will be of no use to her because she has destroyed everything anyway.

The analytic technique as a release of the incorporation of the object

In the analytic technique, it will first be a question of bringing out the incorporates of the object. For Mrs. A., the analytic process will gradually bring to light an identification with her father who also lost forever the woman he loved and was never able to replace her with another love. It is therefore both an incorporative identification with the father abandoned by his mother, a father who waits in vain to find his wife, and another incorporative identification with his abandoning mother: she acted in the same way as his mother did with her partner. On the other hand, it became gradually evident to her that she had blamed her companion for what she had always suffered with her mother, her absence for professional reasons and the fact that she was left alone. We also co-constructed the hypothesis that as a young girl she must have felt guilty about her parents' separation. She regularly repeats: "I cut the link with everyone, I do evil everywhere".

She keeps repeating that she believed that she was the one who was fundamentally destructive but that it relieves her to understand how she carries within her her stepfather who kept devaluing her and was mostly interested in his stepbrothers, not her.

In the course of the analysis, the patient and I will understand that when Mrs. A. says "I'm bad", "it's my fault", she evokes her incorporates of the persecuting father-in-law and of her unavailable mother, who always associates herself with the criticisms of the father-in-law. It is these incorporates that come back to persecute her: for example, when she repeatedly gets angry with her friends, she tries to externalize these persecuting incorporates.

I will link little by little her bonding to her first companion to the bonding to her mother: a transference will take shape on this first companion of the first relation of Mrs. A. to her mother, unattainable, always absent. The transference had in some way already taken place on this companion, before the analysis. Behind incorporative identification, a very archaic form of identification, adhesive identification, emerges: it appears when the child is confronted with an unsatisfactory, disappointing, or even abusive object, which makes separation impossible.

The shadow of the object falls on the act

Shadow on the act

What seemed fundamentally enigmatic to this patient, who said she did not understand herself, was that she had left the apartment where she was living with her partner just when he had agreed to have a baby. The analysis linked this departure to the fact that her mother, who was about to give birth to her first child with her stepfather, had forced her to leave the family home to be housed elsewhere; she was 19 years old. This baby, whom she had always described as an adored little brother, had benefited from all the attention of her parents; a few months later, Mrs. A. suddenly broke up with her mother and her father-in-law who, as a result, had cut her off. In other words, the shadow of the baby had fallen on her act, leaving the shared apartment at the moment when the desired baby with her partner was due to arrive.

Could we say that the shadow of the object has fallen on the act? One can indeed interpret this acting out of her departure precisely at the moment when a baby can arrive as a "representaction" (according to the formulation of J. D. Vincent), that is to say an unconscious representation activated in a hallucinatory way, with motor action: the *agieren* carries here the memory of a trauma.

To free oneself from the splitting between the dark and the ideal side

The analytic process centered on the designation of the incorporates of the object or rather of the objects – here the shadow of the mother, that of the stepfather, that of the baby – allows the patient to free herself from the persecuting shadow, to get out of the splitting between the dark and the ideal side and to be able to face the conflict with the other, tolerating the ambivalence. In general, the analysis of the all-or-nothing processes is essential in the work of extricating the shadow. As far as Mrs. A. is concerned, she gradually stopped disqualifying herself and was able to enter into conflict with the other, without everything being negativized. Her analysis lasted seven years. She was able to emerge from her chronic depression and build a sufficiently happy and balanced life with a husband and children.

"Interpretative reprisals" (J. L. Donnet)

One of the difficulties in the analytic technique consists in not placing the patient on the shadow of a disappointing object, by designating the incorporative identification. I realized in fact that the most unbearable thing for the patients was to think of themselves as identical to a bad incorporated object, so it is preferable to formulate the interventions according to the following modalities: for example, at a moment of the treatment when Mrs. A. feels herself becoming "indifferent, cold and even frozen", according to her own words, "You feel cold and frozen, as you felt at times that your mother was with you ...", emphasizing more the child's experience of deprivation than her identification with a fundamentally disappointing mother .... Or is it possible to say, "Freezing yourself to protect yourself?" and thus emphasize the defense instead of associating the patient with an object without empathy; and the naming of her defense does indeed take her out of the incorporative identification because the object is thus externalized.

The shadow of the patient's object falls on the analyst

Chronic depression often provokes in the analyst a feeling of lassitude, of emptiness and of incompetence in the face of being stuck in repetition. But if the attention is focused on what the patient is making us feel about his or her primary relationship to objects, the session is colored with unsuspected richness. To avoid carrying out interpretative reprisals, according to Jean-Luc Donnet's formula (Donnet & Green, 1973), one of the levers for the analyst is the analysis of his countertransference: it is indeed often the release of his unconscious countertransferential experiences that allows the analyst to spot what the patient has been subjected to in his primary link to the object.

Roussillon (2009) underlined that "What of the object falls on the ego, it is the blind zone of the answer of the object, what the object does not reflect to the subject of itself, there where the object must have function of first mirror". What if the patient could not be welcomed or transformed, comes to the front of the stage and to free itself from the countertransferential opacity represents a first step to seizing the nature of the shadow of the object. The latter reaches the analyst most often in a transference by reversal and it is the analyst's work to treat what could not be treated by the object – what was stopped, petrified and interrupted and therefore what could not unfold its potential.

The shadow of the object falls on the patient's body

I will put forward the hypothesis that one of the specificities of the work of clearing the shadow of the object in the course of an analytic therapy consists in focusing on the way in which the shadow of the object has also fallen on the patient's body. The traumatic characteristics of the first encounter with the object have indeed been inscribed in the primary language of sensorimotor experiences: these archaic experiences will come back in the language of the period in which they were inscribed, in the language of the body and of the act, forms of language that precisely characterize the archaic period, before access to verbal language.

In order to understand the specificity of the analytic work of reviving symbolization processes, I will evoke the example of patients who are very gifted for secondary symbolization, for the play with images and words, but who regularly sink into catastrophic moments where they see everything in black.

Shadow on the body

These patients may, at times, "not feel like they are there anymore", feel like they are "disappearing". They regularly come back from sessions where they collapse, curl up and remain petrified without moving. They say they feel "sucked into the void" or they feel like they are "falling apart", crumbling or becoming "a cloud of dust flying in the air".

In these moments of psychological withdrawal, the patient disappears into hallucinated sensations that could be formulated in the following way:

Shadow on the body (cont.)

"It falls into the void", "it collapses", "it clutches", "it explodes", "it bursts", "it sifts", "it withdraws", "it appears, it disappears", "it exhausts itself", "it disintegrates", "it diffracts", "it shreds", "it nibbles", "it devours", "it turns on itself", "it crushes".

These are formal signifiers, described by Anzieu (1987), bodily impressions that do not belong to the register of fantasy and that impose themselves in the form of hallucinatory experiences. They correspond to proto-representations of space and body – it is a transformation "often felt by the patient as foreign to himself" – which implies a formulation without human subject. This is the reason why the subject is impersonal, "it", or the verb used is reflexive ("it collapses").

The traumatic archaic experiences in the relationship to the object are thus re-actualized in the form of sensory hallucinations. In this context, the analytic technique will consist in linking these sensory impressions, apparently disintegrated from any form of memory, to fragments of memories linked to the object, to "scenic figurations", according to the expression of Aulagnier (1986), in order to try to represent the part of history linked to the object, at the origin of these processes of self-erasing, dusting or diffusion in space.

Shadow on the body (cont.)

I try to link these sensory hallucinations to scenarios related to their history. Thus, for one patient, I first associated his experiences of disappearance, of non-existence with the sudden abandonment of his mother at the age of 4. He then recalled how he used to stay and watch the dust fly in the light, where he would diffract into a thousand pieces. He describes his memory of meals where the adults did not speak to him. He sees himself in front of his toys, unable to play.

Identify the primary forms of symbolization

It is then a question for the analyst of working on the register of primary forms of symbolization (Brun et al., 2014) which engage the body and refer to early experiences. These bodily and sensorimotor experiences appear immobilized by the shadow of the object, in a way petrified, frozen or even decomposed.

The specificity of an analytic listening of the primary forms of symbolization consists in constructing evocative scenes of the relationship to the object from the re-actualization of sensations hallucinated in the patient: thus, according to Aulagnier (1975), to pass from the pictogram to the scenic figuration or fantasy; according to Anzieu (1987), to pass from the formal signifier to the fantasy; according to Bion (1962), from the impersonal 0 to a personal 0, with the ideogram of the protomental. In a general way, it is a question of transforming the perceptive traces, the *fueros*, in representation of a thing, a process that Roussillon names primary symbolization (2009). In this way, the body puts itself little by little into history. The clinical experience shows us that it is the limit and extreme forms of the psychopathology which are particularly solicited in the primary forms of symbolization.

These sensorial/motor forms, therefore, correspond to a hallucinatory return of perceptive traces. Freud will describe in 1937, in "Constructions in analysis", a possible hallucinatory reinvestment *"of something that the child saw or heard at a time when he could hardly speak"* (1937, pp. 278–279, emphasis added). Freud thus brings to the forefront the question of sensory hallucinations in place of recollection. This Freudian conception of hallucination, no longer as the realization of desire on the model of the dream, but as the return in the hallucination of an event of early childhood, allows us to grasp how the shadow of the object can fall on the body, with a possible re-actualization of hallucinated sensations.

I have proposed to name "formal associativity" (Brun, 2019) the associative chain constituted by this emergence of hallucinated sensations, at the same time forms and movements, re-actualizing perceptive traces of archaic experiences linked to the encounter with the object. One of the modalities of access for the analyst to the formal signifiers of the patients consists in listening to their own sensory impressions during the session: what I have proposed to call "shared formal signifiers" appear. Becoming aware of these impressions, which are both corporeal and psychic, allows us to bring these sensory impressions, which are transformed into sensorimotor messages, to figuration, first in the analyst's psyche, then in the dynamics of the analysis. It is also a question of freeing oneself from what Aulagnier (1975) calls the coalescence of the affect and the representation in the pictogram, or Green (1999) calls the indiscrimination between affect and representation: an essential aspect of the cure turns out indeed to be the composition of the affect, from the release of the indistinction between affect and representation in the primary forms of symbolization.

The shadow of the object is not only meant to plunge the subject into negativity; its release can also be a powerful creative resource in the analytical work to reanimate the symbolic potentialities of a subject. This creative potentiality also appeared to me several times at work with artist patients, in the course of their analytic work of releasing the shadow of objects, as much in literary creation as in painting or theater (Brun, 1999). The clinical experience sheds light here on the creative processes at work in artists and vice versa. One of the figures of the creative process haunted by the shadow of the object appears in the work of Thomas Bernhard (1931–89), a contemporary Austrian writer. Thomas Bernhard, evokes his melancholia, in the heart of his writings, as the place where he can always "imagine a dialogue that did not take place, with his brother, his mother":

> It is the dialogue with the past that no longer takes place and will never take place [...] It is the attempt to put one's finger on objects that dissolve at the very moment when one thinks one has touched them.
>
> (2006, p. 33)

Any attempt to touch the shadow of what has not been lived with the objects can only dissolve this shadow forever: writing will be the ultimate attempt to inscribe in the artwork the erasure of the objects and of oneself, to survive it. The artwork stands as a paradoxical commemoration of the shadow of fundamentally disappointing objects. The figure of a shadow of the object not met by the subject emerges here, an object that has not reflected anything of itself to the subject.

But the artwork also feeds on the mad hope to make happen, to deploy, to create finally what did not take place with the object, at the same time loved and hated, and which should have taken place.

References

Anzieu, D. (1987). Les signifiants formels et le moi peau. In: D. Anzieu et al. (Eds.), *Les enveloppes psychiques* (pp. 1–22). Paris: Dunod.

Aulagnier, P. (1975). *La violence de l'interprétation*, Paris: PUF.

Aulagnier, P. (1986). *L'apprenti-historien et le maître-sorcier: Du discours identifiant au discours délirant*. Paris: PUF.

Bernhard, T. (2006). Trois jours. In: *Récits*. Paris: Gallimard, collection Quarto.

Bion, W. R. (1962). *Aux sources de l'expérience*. Paris: PUF, 1979.

Brun, A. (1999). *Henri Michaux ou le corps halluciné, "Les empêcheurs de penser en rond"*. Paris: Seuil.

Brun, A. (2018). *Aux origines du processus créateur*. Ramonville St Agne: Erès, collection Thema-psy.

Brun , A. (2019). *Therapeutic mediations and child psychosis*, 3rd reissue revised and expanded (1st ed. 2007). Paris: Dunod.

Brun, A., Roussillon, R. et al. (2014). *Les formes primaires de symbolisation*. Paris: Dunod.

Donnet, J-L., & Green, A. (1973). *L'enfant de ça*. Paris: Éditions de Minuit.

Freud, S. (1914). Pour introduire le narcissisme, trans. J. Laplanche. Paris, Gallimard, 1968; *OCF-P*, XII 1913–1914, 2005, pp. 213–245, *GW*, X.

Freud, S. (1917e [1915]). Mourning and melancholia, *Metapsychology*, trans. J. Laplanche, J-B. Pontalis, J-P. Briand, J-P. Grossein, & M. Tort. Paris: Gallimard, 1968; *OCF-P*, XIII: 261–280, 1988; *GW*, X.

Freud, S. (1921). Psychology of the masses and analysis of the self, trans. by J. Altounian, A. Bourguignon, & P. Cotet, *OCF-P*, XVI: 1–83, 1991; *GW*, XIII.

Freud, S. (1923b). Le moi et le ça, *Essais de psychanalyse*, trans. J. Laplanche, *OCF.P*, XVI: 255–301; 1991, *GW*, XIII.

Freud, S. (1937d). Constructions in analysis, *Results, ideas, problems*, II, trans. E. R. Hawelka, U. Huber, & J. Laplanche. Paris: PUF, 1985; *GW*, XVI.

Green, A. (1999). On discrimination and indiscrimination affect-representation. *Revue française de psychanalyse*, 1999, t. LXIII(1), 217–271.

McDougall, J. (1982). *Théâtres du JE*. Paris: Galllimard.

Michaux, H. (1963). La ralentie, OC, T1, *La Pléiade*, 573–580.

Roussillon, R. (2009). La transmission et la conversation primitive. In: M. Sassolas (Ed.), *Transmissions et soins psychiques* (pp. 47–55). Ramonville St Agne: Erès.

Roussillon, R. (2019). La fonction de l'objet dans la symbolisation et la désymbolisation. In: A. Brun, B. Chouvier, & S. Roussillon (Eds.), *Symbolisation et environnements* (pp. 11–32). Paris: Dunod.

9   Together in the magma of despair

Valérie Bouville

Both described analyses concern patients with severe chronic depression. In the first case, multiple traumatization in childhood is manifest. In the second case, in the course of treatment, it turns out that the patient grew up in someone else's shadow. The text is devoted to the intensive transference–countertransference interaction in analytic treatment.

As a young child, Ms. B had to leave her life to flee the civil war that had suddenly started in her home country. Her father being a military man actively involved in the fighting, her mother, then in the last stages of pregnancy with the youngest of her siblings, was left alone with her young children to walk across the country. A long and dangerous march, during which Ms. B suffered at least one trauma of which she has images and sounds, led them hundreds of kilometres to a quieter region where her mother's family lived, whom she had not known until then. After a few days, Ms. B's mother left her with her family before continuing her journey to Germany, taking only her young sons with her. After what would have been a very long time even for an adult, she arranged for her daughter to come to Germany, and Ms. B flew there unaccompanied. On arrival in Germany, Ms. B learned that her father had died two years earlier.

When she first came to see me, she had been living in Germany for several decades. She told me that her main problem was that she systematically gave up on everything she started and could not see how to continue her life. After a steady decline in her performance in high school, she had been transferred to a school for very low-achieving students and had struggled to obtain her middle school diploma. Since then, unskilled jobs, which she could only hold for a short period of time, alternated with longer and longer periods of unemployment, during which she had to "recover". The unemployment services had offered her numerous training courses, which she had started and then stopped after a few weeks for no understandable reason. There was actually no reason for this, Ms. B explained to me: "Everything was going well, but one day I did not go there anymore".

At our first appointment, Ms. B told me that I was the third therapist she had seen, the previous ones having explained that they could not help her. I had been recommended to her by the health service as a war specialist and, as

DOI: 10.4324/9781003279297-9

I wondered in surprise where I had got this reputation, she was in fact indirectly communicating what was probably the most important piece of information from the first meeting: she had come from the war, hoped I would get over the shock, but expected to be sent away again. In fact, the decision of the colleagues before me seemed quite understandable, as Ms. B was clearly communicating the feeling that dealing with her would be a waste of time.

The interpersonal dynamics of this first encounter were impressive in that Ms. B was sending a double message, something like "Please take me" and "What do you want from me?" These two messages acted as two agonistic and antagonistic forces which, when used with a slight time lag, only allow the beginning of a movement to be stopped dead in its acceleration phase and ultimately prevent any movement at all. This phenomenon had spread to me, probably by projective identification, so that it was only after she had left and after I had regained some mental mobility that I understood what had just happened. I assumed then that these agonistic–antagonistic forces were responsible for the symptom she had presented to me as her reason for treatment: when she started something, such as a reintegration (agonistic) program, the antagonistic force would mobilize and increase until she gave up. I had the impression from the start that both forces had good reason to exist.

I proposed to Ms. B, whom I found, beyond her extinct and impoverished appearance, beautiful, intelligent and emotionally rich, an analytical treatment that would allow us on the one hand to have enough time to explore her multiple traumatic history, and on the other hand to understand the two paralysing forces individually, in their bijective dynamics and in all their effects.

After a few months of treatment, during which Ms. B's speech had gradually turned into logorrhea and had made our contact increasingly difficult, she first cancelled several appointments and then stopped the treatment by informing me by phone. This manifestation of her main symptom, abandoning everything she started, was not very surprising, but it triggered in me a deep anguish of dissolution. A horrible feeling of abandonment and endless waiting for another who might never come back came over me. I thought of the little girl who had been abandoned and then suspected that the second force "What do you want from me?" was there to protect her from being abandoned again by the object by pushing it away herself before it became too important. She had to maintain her hold on the object.

After a few weeks she contacted me again, first by sending me a Christmas card and then by calling to ask how I was. Surprised, I responded politely but distantly to her call and it was only after I hung up that I realized she was probably calling for help. So I sent her a card in return for her card and offered her a meeting, which she immediately accepted. We resumed our analytical work, both enriched by this essential unconscious message. This was the last time she interrupted a project, resuming the course of training she had abandoned as a teenager until she obtained a professional qualification and finally a permanent job. If this short sentence should give the impression that the path was easy, I must add that the analytical path was full of uncertainties, many moments of imminent destruction and fruitless desert crossings. The treatment lasted about ten years.

I would like to mention here two elements of the treatment that I think enabled Ms. B to give up her main symptom. First, and this seems to me to be the main element in her readiness to move again, she found in the analyst a usable object in the sense that Winnicott understands it:

> This sequence can be observed: (1) Subject relates to object. (2) Object is in process of being found instead of placed by the subject in the world. (3) Subject destroys object. (4) Object survives destruction. (5) Subject can use object. The object is always being destroyed. This destruction becomes the unconscious backcloth for love of a real object; that is, an object outside the area of the subject's omnipotent control.
>
> (Winnicott, 1969, p. 714)

The second tangible element that I would like to mention consists of a phenomenon that I will now describe in more detail and that was decisive in our analytical/therapeutic interaction: the logorrheic defence that occurred before the abandonment of the treatment a few weeks after its beginning manifested itself repeatedly during the treatment. During her long monologues, which kept me at a distance and did not allow any intervention or reflection on my part, verbal and averbal elements continued to appear, reminding me after very long minutes of psychic emptiness within me of some of the small amount of information I had about her early childhood. Images and sketchy connections between the here and now and her memories from earlier sessions would appear to me. Sometimes the incubation period, the aforementioned desert, lasted several weeks and the listening tested my patience. It was exhausting, but also hopeless, and I finally asked myself: "What's the point?", one of Ms. B's guiding principals ("*Leitmotive*").

I had become Ms. B, in the sense that Bion (1965) means when he talks about "becoming". I was bogged down, without a future, without light, a failing energy vaporized in a repetitive movement in extinction ... I then drew the only card I had in my pocket as one clutches at a straw: I formulated the images and connections just mentioned as a hypothesis. To my astonishment Ms. B stopped at the interpretation and got in touch with me again (according to Bion's categories of interpretation, an interpretation of attention). For example: "The atmosphere here at the moment reminds me of the situation you mentioned about your long walk, when you refused to continue and your mother got angry".

I could not say whether these interpretations were correct or not, i.e. whether or not they took up what Ms. B was unconsciously trying to convey to me, because they were my images and appeared to me to be cleaved from Ms. B's discourse. What is certain, however, is that they offered a way out of the lack of perspective and led to new memories, new images and new feelings of the buried past. In the long run, they allowed the constitution of a narrative of her story.

Since her arrival in Germany, Ms. B had not heard anything about her home country, about her previous life. Her mother tongue was replaced by German. Her mother did not speak from there. While the world around her was becoming more stable, part of her inner world was closing in on itself. Memories of her previous life gradually faded to the point where she lost all conscious awareness of them, while she remained fixated on a sense of lost paradise linked to her father. At the beginning of the treatment, she was full of reproaches towards her mother who had taken her from her paradise and left her with strangers before taking her away again to an even stranger country. Unconsciously, she blamed her mother for killing her father by leaving him behind when she fled, while Ms. B continued to remain faithful to him by not going any further. The antagonistic force mentioned several times and active between us from the first meeting was partly based on this unconscious desire: to stop the progressive movement away from the beloved object, to stop time by immobility in order to prevent the loss of the past and the destruction of the link to the beloved object. Discovering this has given us part of the explanation for his symptoms, organized in unconscious offshoots that are cleaved from each other. The description of the Horcruxes in the last part of the Harry Potter saga (*Harry Potter and the Deathly Hallows*, Rowling, 2007) seems to me to illustrate the disarticulation and separation of the elements constituting the unconscious pathological mechanism, which can only be translated and disarmed when all the elements and their mnemonic traces are gathered and understood in their articulation.

During the course of the analysis and in parallel with the gradual reappearance of her memories, Ms. B reconnected with her mother, who in turn began to talk about their country of origin and their past. As their exchanges intensified, Ms. B realized that her mother had banished the past, her language and her country of origin from their emotional and family life because these memories were too painful for her. She had hoped to give her children the opportunity to "forget and start again".

Following her mother's tacit expectation, Ms. B had blocked the past within her; at the same time and against her mother's hope, she had also made a mausoleum of this past whose extinctive flame she kept permanently active. I refer here to André Green's description of the mausoleum in "The Dead Mother" (Green, 1980) and Bernard Chervet's description of the extinctive regressive drive tendency in "Pulses, do you have a life?" (Chervet, 2014).

The fact that I wanted to know about this past and considered it valuable had at first surprised Ms. B. She then felt an unexpected revaluation of her person that was completely contrary to her self-image. For years Ms. B had been subjecting herself to the inner racism that Fahkry Davids (Davids, 2016) talks about. Through introspective identification with the external white role models around her, she rejected a part of herself out of racism while externally struggling against the racism she was exposed to on a daily basis. Here we discovered a new part of the explanation (another Horcrux) of the agonist–antagonist mechanism, i.e. of her symptom.

An essential instrument in the treatment of this chronic depression was the systematic, albeit not linear, reconstruction of the traumatic history. In his work on trauma patients, Werner Bohleber emphasizes the importance of revealing the reality of the trauma (Bohleber, 2012). Ms. B constantly doubted the veracity of her memories, or rather she remained uncertain about the reality of her memories.

In her family, under the rule of silence, she had not had access to exchanges, comparisons and confirmations of her perceptions of situations, atmospheres, interactions by family members and did not trust what she perceived. As is often the case with psychotics, Ms. B could not trust her perception and spent endless hours stuck in thought loops about whether something was true or not. The gradual reintegration during treatment of the cleaved fragments of self began with the emergence of the memory and continued with the repetitive external confirmation – in this case by the analyst – of its reality. It was through confirmation by the object that the disorganized and blurred mnemonic fragments became tangible memories capable of aligning themselves into a transformative narrative.

The second vignette I would now like to discuss concerns the treatment of chronic depression accompanied by more or less acute suicidal thoughts. Mr. A is young, lives abroad, does not speak the language of the country in which he lives and uses a third language at work.

He came to see me on the advice of his girlfriend and explained that he was having a lot of trouble making up his mind. He told me that he could spend hours trying to formulate a written sentence without succeeding, turning the words over and over in his head. He was thinking all the time without being able to act. Every subject, every decision to come, no matter how insignificant, made him think in great detail about the possible consequences of a decision. He would remain inhibited for hours or even days, eventually making a decision which he would immediately regret and which would lead him to despair.

The decision for an analytical treatment was, in comparison, quite easy to take. The fact that this decision involved both of us played an essential role, I think.

The analysis was characterized by a marked inhibition caused by the compulsive defence described above.

Mr. A showed little inclination to free association from the outset, as his intellectual defence, like a censor, rejected almost any idea. He would then silently or loudly ponder philosophical ideas in a monotone of dull contempt. The interpretations offered, whether simple summaries, reflections or descriptions of mechanisms, were systematically deconstructed and then rejected as inadequate or systematically confirmed but without progressive effect. He remained at a distance, as if behind a black opaque wall. He systematically arrived late, only setting off for the practice when the session was supposed to start. After a few months he began to describe his procrastination in writing work letters, which he did not write, took home and continued not to write in his free time. He would stall, put himself out of time while seeing time around him move forward and blame himself for his inefficiency. The sessions remained empty of life but full of a nagging complaint. Mr. A only brought to the sessions damning reflections on his inability to be coherent in his work. My invitations to talk about the rest of his life, in which things were obviously happening, marriage, family exchanges, visits, remained ignored. We didn't seem to be allowed to go off topic. Over the months I gradually realized that instead of the sessions relieving Mr. A, they were actually starting me. The oil slick in which he was living was gradually invading me. When I interpreted this, cautiously, for fear of making him feel guilty, he reacted promptly by saying that he had always been afraid of hurting others, that he wanted to protect others from him and from all the bad that was in him. The next day he brought the first dream, describing a dark labyrinth keeping him prisoner as he tried relentlessly but in vain to find his way out. The atmosphere of the dream was both eerie and familiar, dark, cold, but known. While Mr. A had "no association" I saw the labyrinth from above and thought that it would be enough to rise to get out of it … The Minotaur came to mind, symbol of animality and the dominance of the impulses, as well as Theseus, managing to kill him by trickery. I thought that Mr. A was both the Minotaur and Theseus. This dream gave a first summary in images of his compulsive and failing superego and of his helpless and hopeless self. I interpreted with him the labyrinthine constellation between us: he as the tormented ego, I as the tormented superego, and vice versa. For the first time after almost a year of treatment, a first psychic relief was felt. We understood that he unconsciously refused to leave this "labyrinth" in which he felt trapped and which seemed to him to have no way out, in order to tackle other subjects. He unconsciously forbade himself any lively and fruitful relationship. The Minotaur was dangerous, monstrous and should not be allowed out. Although the resemblance between this superego and his succinct description of the family atmosphere of his childhood was obvious, he rejected the comparison strongly. The relief was only temporary, and a negative therapeutic reaction followed, with many more hours of procrastination.

The treatment continued like this: many hours of procrastination, suddenly an hour of clarity where Mr. A became accessible with a psychodynamically relevant discovery and then procrastination again. He seemed to have completely forgotten the previous day's discovery by the next session (like the patient presented by Bernard Reith, Chapter 6 in this volume).

He then began to complain about the "sectarian, dogmatic" analytical method and his lying down situation, while I took him from above and behind, and then to criticize me directly, rather nastily but still without raising the tone of his usual monotone. At the same time his situation on the outside seemed to be improving. If Mr. A didn't notice it himself, others did. He was getting better. He didn't know if he should be grateful to me or not, after all I wasn't doing much …

While I seriously doubted my ability to help him and my analytical abilities at all, a growing desire to respond to his denigrating attacks with verbal jousts made me fear that I was about to act out. These particularly painful aggressive impulses seemed to me both perfectly justified and completely unacceptable but also very alien to me. I felt on the verge of an explosion and, after a long internal *procrastination* during which he continued a monotone monologue, tried to interpret them based on the idea of projective identification (cf. Melanie Klein). Something like: "I wonder if you are angry. The atmosphere today seems particularly tense". He stopped his monologue and then opened up for the first time about the more or less virulent obsessive thoughts and images that had been accompanying him constantly since adolescence and that regularly flared up during the sessions: they were images of bloody aggressions against himself that were extremely violent and systematically led to his death, demanded by a superego mad with hatred against him and insulting him relentlessly. The sharing of these images with me, at first hesitant and sporadic, became on my repeated invitation little by little possible at the time they occurred during the session, allowing me to finally recognize the first part of the trigger: an interpretation, sometimes anodyne, touching him. The irruption of violent images blocked the emotional effects of the interpretation and interrupted our contact. This very effective defence cancelled out the interpretation and the associations that had led us to it, as well as any potential new associations.

Shortly after this change in the sessions Mr. A began, after repeatedly telling me that they were untouchable and that he would not let me sully their image, to describe his parents' lifelong conflict and his helpless desire for it to end. But above all he didn't want to burden them (and on that he was able to act). He also began to talk about another member of the family, his lifelong idol, whose playmate he had been, but also the whipping boy throughout his childhood.

To come to the sharing of his violent obsessive thoughts he had to go through a common labyrinth in which the analyst had to join him and had first become his sufferer, companion of despair and alter ego. It was from within this common melancholic space, this "melancholia for two" as Jean-Claude Rolland called it in the discussion that followed the presentation of this paper, that the countertransference revealed the hatred against a beloved object, essential to psychic existence, a violent, bloody, murderous hatred that was absolutely forbidden and turned on the ego, this object of identification whose "shadow [had] fallen on the ego" (Freud, 1917, p. 435).

The sharing of his obsessive thoughts was an important step in the treatment of Mr. A. He had let me enter little by little into his melancholic world (the oil slick), then communicated by projective identification his anger, his hatred but also his restraint against the object, communication in the form of projected beta fragments (cf. Bion, 1965). The analyst's work then consisted in gathering and analysing these fragments while defusing their intrinsic submerging affects (alpha function, cf. Bion, 1965) before reformulating them into a bearable interpretation that finally allowed him to open up from his torturing thoughts.

The treatment, still ongoing at the time of my writing, then went through a long phase that I would describe as adolescence. Mr. A seemed to catch up in the analysis with the internal and external conflict of puberty that he had not experienced in adolescence. To be able to attack the object (in this case the analyst) without fearing a collapse on the part of the analyst or himself was an essential condition for this stage of emancipation. I understood to what extent his family members, whom he placed above the common people and whose superior intellectual and emotional intelligence he praised, appeared to him in the end so fragile that he had not been able to *use* them in Winnicott's sense. His distrust of the adults of his parents' generation had at first seemed surprising to me and was now explained.

The interpretation of her identification with these objects has not yet been possible and here I would like to take up the technical advice given by Anne Brun in Chapter 8 in this volume: be careful not to name the object identification if it reinforces the hatred against oneself. The mechanism described by Freud in "Mourning and Melancholia" (Freud, 2017) of turning hatred towards a disappointing object of identification and the unconscious disinvestment of that object against the own ego was, of course, active when Mr. A first came to see me in the midst of a severe depression. The object involved was no longer the same as that of his adolescence, but the mechanism he had developed in the past remained the only means available to him to cope with the internalized conflict with this beloved and disappointing object. Our gradual approach to the source of his unhappiness critically reinforced the mechanism and a very worrying suicidal period began as my summer holidays approached. I was faced with a technical dilemma: to interpret what I understood, to name the object, or to abstain and wait impatiently, or even to propose a hospitalization? I asked Mr. A to wait until I returned, not to do anything until we understood more. Mr. A promised and he held firm. When the sessions resumed he read me what he had written during my absence. His detailed description of the suicide he had prepared and acted upon up to the fateful moment, which he had finally renounced, thinking of the object that would not recover, made me waver inside, and that is an understatement. I think it was good not to name the object, as if to lance the abscess, before the holiday interruption for fear that he would act out (suicidally). In writing, Mr. A opted to maintain the link, he relied on the internal framework that remained in place despite my absence and he himself recognized the object, even if he did not yet perceive the extent of its harmful unconscious hold.

We still have a long way to go before the reconstruction of the unconscious mechanism at the origin of his melancholy can be recognized and interpreted in its entirety, but Mr. A is better, he is no longer suicidal; life and himself seem to him at this moment worthy of respect and longevity.

Of these two psychoanalytic treatments of chronic depression, one resulted from several childhood traumas, the other without any obvious trauma or loss that could explain the depression externally. The treatment of these pathologies is long and painstaking, fraught with discouragement, misunderstandings and dangers that put both patient and analyst to a severe test. I think I can say that it is always worthwhile.

References

Bion, W. R.(1965/ 1984). *Transformations*. London:Routledge.

Bohleber, W. (2012). Was Psychoanalyse heute leistet. Identität und Intersubjektivität. *Trauma und Therapie, Gewalt und Gesellschaft*. Stuttgart: Klett-Cotta-Verlag.

Green, A. (1980). The dead mother. In: *Narcissism of life, narcissism of death* (1983). Paris: Editions de Minuit.

Chervet, B. (2014). Pulsions, avez-vous une vie? *Revue française de psychosomatique*, 1(45), 103–128.

Davids, F. (2016). *Innerer Rassismus*. Gießen: Psychosozial-Verlag.

Freud, S. (1917). Trauer und Melancholie, *GW Band X*. Frankfurt am Main: Fischer Taschenbuch Verlag, p. 435.

Rowling, J. K. (2007). *Harry Potter and the deathly hallows*. London: Arthur A. Levine Books.

Winnicott, D. W. (1969). The use of an object. *International Journal of Psychoanalysis*, 50, 711–716.

10 The presence of God in a melancholic patient

Gérard Winterhalter

"It's the end of my life." It was at the age of 11, when he was placed in a foster home, that this patient stated for himself what was at first a particularly intense experience. His parents could only visit him once a month. His mother and father were in constant conflict, even in front of their children. Domestic scenes lasted well into the night. The patient tried unsuccessfully to stop the shouting. Two years later, his parents divorced for good. "I closed my heart forever", he says. He still hoped to return to his family. At the foster home, the director enforced order through fear, violence and beatings. The only outings allowed were to a Christian movement, where cultural and sports activities took his mind off things. In this gloomy picture, two elements were happier: (a) The patient had better results at school than the other residents; (b) A love story, forbidden by the headmaster, with a young girl from the foster home gave him a new taste for life.

When he finished his compulsory schooling, he returned to live with his father. He went to business school, found work in banking. Later he got married, had no children, got divorced and lost his job. He found other jobs, and then was again fired, with a feeling of injustice. He tried to have other relationships. Not easy. He travelled several times to rebuild his professional and emotional life, and contacted me upon his return from the last of these trips. He was beaten up in a fight in an unclear context, which generated a new psychological trauma that left him exhausted.

This patient of about 50 years of age thus arrives at his first consultation, three years ago now. He presents himself with anxieties that quickly turn to panic about his future, and severe depressive symptoms. He has concentration problems and loses his memory. He sleeps badly. He has always had very little pleasure in life, and this is more intense now. He has never had any self-confidence or self-esteem. He has always tried to adapt as best as he could by bowing his head. He needs to be believed, since the beginning of his life, and I feel this very strongly in the way he tells me things.

The atmosphere of the session is heavy, an infinite sadness can be read on his face, he is prostrated on his armchair. An intense distressing experience is palpable, and the need for reassurance is marked. He is very lonely, in spite of some old acquaintances that he contacts from time to time and his brother,

DOI: 10.4324/9781003279297-10

with whom the link alternates between complicity and conflicts. I immediately feel a sense of despair, a despair that I know is partly the patient's own, but in which I also perceive that something of my own melancholic core is at work. I didn't expect this, and I wondered how much I could take. I gradually got back on track during the interview. It is a question of containing this first inner defensive movement, and recovering the first positive feelings that I had had on the phone when he had asked to be admitted to consult.

A double listening is set up, a medical listening and a psychoanalytical listening. I am familiar with this double listening, as I worked for a long time in an emergency and crisis centre. The work of crisis consists in starting from the conflicts between the patient and his external reality in order to progressively reach the awareness of an internal conflictuality, which has remained unconscious until then. It becomes possible to build the indication for a psychoanalytic psychotherapy, or even for an analytic cure (de Coulon, 2021; Despland et al., 2010).

From a medical point of view, considering the clinic presentation and in particular my own inner experience, the first thing is to make sure that this patient stays alive, that he will be able to face his own destructiveness. He tells me that he is ready for God to come and get him, but that he does not have the courage to kill himself, and that he has no intention of hurting others. Sometimes he prays and reads texts from the Bible, which allows him to bear being alive. I note that God has remained present for him, in a protective way. Normally, the child does not have to prove that he exists and that he has a place for his parents. Here, I begin to think that he vitally needs a place where he is accepted as he is. Indeed, this patient has put himself throughout his life in an adaptive position to correspond to what was expected of him, or what he believes was expected of him. His explicit request is that I protect him and do something for him. This is the first time he is consulting with a psychiatrist; he has no preconceived idea of what a psychiatric and psychotherapeutic treatment consists of. "What I can do is listen to you", I tell him. He agreed to come for two sessions a week in a traditional setting for one-on-one psychoanalytic psychotherapy. Any medication was prescribed by his family doctor. We also discussed the possibilities of help in case of emergency, if he could no longer manage possible suicidal impulses. Over the three years of his treatment, he arrived punctually at all his sessions.

During the first half of this psychotherapy, I primarily listen to him talking about his current suffering. The main complaint that emerges is that nothing is given to him, that he has always had to fight to be accepted, and that he is exhausted by this. This situation is going to strain my endurance. The atmosphere remains heavy, and the sessions burdensome. There are few signs of improvement. I have the feeling that he is now waiting for someone to give him good news, without being able to say what good news would be for him, or where it might come from. I inevitably show, because it is a basic position that I personally hold, a certain benevolence and a rather active position if necessary. In other words, I assume a position of presence in withdrawal rather than a withdrawal of presence, to use the title of an article by the French psychoanalyst Dominique Bourdin devoted to this theme (Bourdin, 2007). This is particularly the case in this situation, where I take the decision to position myself, at first, as a "*Nebenmensch*", as a helping object. Most of the time, it is possible for me to move from a benevolence that is as neutral as possible to a neutrality that remains tinged with a little benevolence, as the patient appropriates the therapeutic space proposed to develop an affective play and a freer associativity. Here, I notice that it does not progress.

Questions emerge: Is there hope in this situation? Who is carrying this hope? What are the implications for further psychotherapy? I realize that my mind is numb, lazy, and that I am experiencing mostly a sense of weariness. I am looking for help in a supervision group. One of the major interests of this type of group supervision is that it allows for associations and daydreams to be encouraged and thus to restore a space of thinking. I kept from the supervision that it is a question of getting out of my overly benevolent position and finding an opportunity to interpret the patient's aggression in the transference. In other words, too much empathy kills empathy. Perhaps most importantly, through the associations of the group, I have regained a liveliness of thought.

Initially, I seized opportunities in the patient's discourse to co-construct a richer narrative of his story. Here are some brief elements of his father: He would first say that he just had to obey him; later, he mentioned that his father had shared his interest in history and geography with him. As for his mother, she told him that he should never be too happy. It is, nevertheless, she who gave him a good education. His brother, seven years younger than him, was luckier – he had a strong character, said the patient, and achieved more than he did and was more adaptable. The patient regretted having to leave the foster home and the Christian movement to return to live with his father at 17. It was the only place where he had finally integrated and made friends.

His love life was poor. The wife he had was too authoritarian, and he briefly dated a few other women. He now has a girlfriend, with whom he has a friendly relationship rather than a romantic one. This is enough for him. I have now learned that in his forties, after his divorce, he reconnected with the Christian group he had felt comfortable with during his teenage years. This time, he invested more in the religious dimension of the group. He found the human warmth that he missed so much, and his suffering made sense. According to this movement, if one suffered, it meant that one was truthful. The patient also participated in the exaltation present in religious ceremonies, and felt he had a family. Gradually, however, following the strict rules of the movement became too difficult for him. He felt that he was returning to the straitjacket imposed by both his foster home and his father. The freedom that the group had given him in his adolescence was no longer there. He then left the movement, this time of his own account, and began to travel until his last attack.

After two years of psychotherapy, he was doing better. The patient wanted to work again. However, attempts to find a job, and then various measures of unemployment insurance to try to reintegrate him, failed. He finally obtained a pension for his disability. This time, the society was giving him something. He was aware of this, he needed it. On the other hand, it was hard for him to accept this, he who had worked so hard to find a place in society, to remain independent. He was waiting for something else. I told him that maybe he was also expecting something else from me, and that he was angry with me for not giving it to him. At first, he said that he was not angry with me. Later, he said that he expected more warmth from me, that I am too intellectual. I told him that it was a good thing he could be angry – it often helps in a situation like his. The interruption of the sessions for vacations provided further opportunities to work on aggressiveness in the transference. Before each vacation period, he gradually asks more of his girlfriend; he wants her to be closer, he wants them to have a relationship other than a friendly one. He has romantic feelings for her, which surprises him. The girlfriend, however, wants to maintain the existing relationship; but this relationship turns stormy.

I tell the patient that he seems more attached to me and that he now suffers from my absences. This has a calming effect. But he remains very questionable about the attachment he might have to me. It is the repetition of these relational movements with his friend and their interpretation that will gradually allow the patient to become aware of the internal ambivalence he has about me. As time goes by, he associates more easily. At one point, he recalls the catechism classes he had taken as a child, his curiosity for the commentaries on the texts of the Bible and his attachment to the pastor who gave these classes. This pastor was warm towards him, he took him under his wing. Already at the age of 15, he had entrusted him with catechism classes to give to the younger children. All this stopped at 17 when he had to return to live with his father. I realize that for a few years he was able to be in contact with a benevolent father figure. That said, what interested me most at that time was his curiosity for biblical texts. I was then reminded of a reading by Florence Guignard that articulates epistemophilic drive and masochism (Guignard, 2015).

I am interested in this curiosity. I notice an openness in this patient, who tells me about his thirst for knowledge, which was on the whole suppressed by his father, who forced him to go to business school rather than to study. We briefly engage in a dialogue around certain biblical texts. A desire to study theology emerges in the patient. This is the first time I see hope in him. I share and support both this desire and this hope. I feel it was important not to miss this opportunity, being convinced that the patient would not go any further on his own, and that masochism would take over. Eventually, he enrols in part-time Bible classes at a private school. He wants to study, to succeed in his studies, and to disprove the place his father had assigned him. The first year of classes is hard for him, hard to get used to the place, hard to meet new people, hard to start studying. But he realizes that he likes taking classes, that he is in the right place. He knows he needs more time than others, but he enjoys reading, learning more about what has been said, learning well. He finally is able to make connections with new people.

A new hardship came at the end of winter 2019–20. This was the closing of all schools due to the pandemic. Classes are held via video conferencing. The patient does not leave his home. His girlfriend keeps more distance from him than he would like. He finds himself very lonely. The depressive symptoms become more prominent, as does the masochism. It is as if his father was right, he is not made to study. At the same time, anger gradually emerges. He is not given an easy task, nothing is given to him, he is still the one who has to fight and he wants to give up everything. Even if I feel slightly the address of this anger in the transference, without his being able to formulate clearly to me what it is about, I opt to focus my interventions on the curiosity which has been present until now. These interventions give him back some hope, and he starts to study again.

A first series of exams takes place in June; he successfully passes three out of four. He is happy, but blames himself for having panicked on the fourth one, it reminds him of his father's comments on his incapacity, and he loses confidence again. This continues during the summer with my absence. When I come back, he feels cold all the time, as if he is refrigerated, and nothing and nobody can warm him up. He doesn't even have the strength to be angry with me anymore. The resumption of the sessions allows a slight appeasement. He speaks to me again about the Christian movement, the warmth he found there, the exaltation that allowed him to feel the presence of God. He thinks he would find some aspects of this in the study of the texts of the Bible, but it does not work, because what is taught in this school is a critical study of the texts. Something broke. This is not a new observation, but it is resurfacing. He is going to start studying again. He is very anxious at the idea of failing a second time the exam he has to retake. My voice is reassuring – the patient seems to know the material well. In the session that follows this exam, for the first time, he makes a balanced and, in my opinion, relevant assessment of what had happened. In the first part of the exam, where he had to answer questions, he did well, which gave him confidence. In the second part, he realized when he left the room, when nothing could be changed, that he had not read the instructions correctly, and that he had only done half of the work required. Anguish overcame him; he wrote a message to the expert to try to prove his good faith. During the session, he is devastated, but also really angry. He blames himself and realizes that he has no one to blame but himself. He asks me if this can happen unconsciously. I tell him that it can happen.

He takes up the rhetoric of the Christian movement he had attended, which valued suffering because it meant that one was on the right track. Now he cannot stand suffering any longer, especially since he realizes in a new way that he is the one who is feeding this suffering, in relation to what has made him happy during this year. I am a little disconcerted by the strength of this anger, which this time is not plaintive anger. I just manage to tell him that he has certainly been able to perceive that the Bible was full of conflicts, and that a careful reading could also help him to perceive how God, and then Jesus, dealt with these conflicts. That it could perhaps help him to see what he wants to do with his own, now that he has a better perception of the internal psychological dimension of them.

While writing on these sessions, I am also reflecting on how to interpret this anger in the transference. I think back to the God guarantor of his survival in the early days of psychotherapy, and I realize that the patient gradually invested me in the same way. He gradually became convinced that he had a place in my consultation as he was. This confidence came in connection with the establishment of a good-enough relationship, also including the interpretation in the transference of the first movements of anger that he could address to me. Now another God appears, that of his second passage in the Christian movement. An exalting God, certainly, but also a God who assigns to a given place and who values suffering. I thus became this God, the idealized father the patient is unable to mourn. My interest in his curiosity, my support of his decision to return to school, with the note of hope that this decision carries, certainly contributed to this modality of investment in the transference. In other words, I have carried too much of a desire, a longing, in the patient's place, and I can feel that he needs to disengage from that. "Before killing the Oedipal father, it is a question of doing the work of the death of the ideal father." These words, attributed to Pierre Fédida, which I was reminded of in supervision recently about another situation, ring particularly true at this moment. They will certainly inspire the work to come, but also the disengagement that I have to make by positioning myself now more in the background and in a position more marked by neutrality.

At the end of this chapter, here are some more general thoughts:

The work of Werner Bohleber and Marianne Leuzinger Bohleber (2016) on the specificities of interpretive work in the treatment of traumatized patients is very enlightening in this situation: they postulate the necessity of building a secure bond before being able to approach the actualization of the traumatic experience. This presupposes a certain quality of presence, with particular attention to not inducing a regression that would quickly prove to be unbearable and potentially dangerous. This is what seems to have happened here, the patient having gradually acquired a feeling of internal security thanks to the stability and reliability of the proposed therapeutic relationship. As this sense of security developed, it became possible to address some dimensions of the internal traumatic experience and its unconscious repercussions in the patient's approach to relationships. We arrived at an actualization of this experience in the transference, admittedly partial, but bringing hope for the continuation of this psychotherapy.

Another element which, in my opinion, contributes to the improvement of the state of health of these patients is the active interest shown by the therapist in what may have made them curious in their childhood and youth. The reunion with the epistemophilic drive that animates all life will help to make the mortifying masochism give way to a greater or lesser extent, as we know that it also serves to maintain the phantasmatic illusion of fusion with a good object.

One more word about the question of God's presence in this patient: It is not difficult to realize how indispensable the presence of an external God was to his survival. As the psychotherapy progressed, the image of this God evolved, as much in connection with the co-construction of the patient's history as with the evolution of the transference and countertransference dynamic, which found there a favourable place to lateralize. It will be interesting to follow, in this situation, to what extent the need for an external God will be maintained and, if necessary, if it will be possible for this God to serve more the reconstruction of the ego than its alienation (de Saussure, 2009).

References

Bohleber, W. & Leuzinger-Bohleber, M. (2016). The special problem of interpretation in the treatment of traumatized patients. *Psychoanalytic Inquiry*, 36(1), 60–76.

Bourdin, D. (2007). Pour une présence en retrait qui ne soit pas un retrait de présence. Note sur l'altérité de l'analyste. *Revue Française de Psychanalyse*, 71(3), 719–738.

De Coulon, N. (2021). *La crise, stratégies d'intervention thérapeutique en psychiatrie*, 2nd ed. Paris: Antipodes.

De Saussure, T. (2009). *L'inconscient, nos croyances et la foi chrétienne. Etudes psychanalytiques et bibliques*. Paris: Cerf.

Despland, J. N., Michel, L., & de Roten, Y. (2010). *Intervention psychodynamique brève, un modèle de consultation thérapeutique chez l'adulte*. Paris: Elsevier Masson.

Guignard, F. (2015). *Quelle psychanalyse pour le XXIème siècle. Tome 1, Concepts psychanalytiques en mouvement*. Paris: Editions Ithaque.

11 Some aspects of early development and depression

The case of Thea, an adolescent

Silke Kratel Cañellas

The first psychoanalysts dealt with adults, constructing hypotheses about the child their patients had been, working on psychic conflicts linked to infantile sexuality. Children were not taken into psychotherapy or psychoanalysis at that time. Today, psychoanalysis and psychotherapy of the child is widely practised, enlightened in particular by research on the development of the child and the adolescent. In Geneva, we have been lucky enough to have many internationally renowned teachers, researchers and psychoanalysts who have contributed to the birth and development of this discipline that I must renounce naming them all here for lack of space.

In 1995, Palacios Espasa and Dufour wrote that for a long time depression in children was not recognized as such because its manifestations differ from those of adults. Depression in children and adolescents rarely manifests itself as sadness or despondency. The child becomes rather inhibited, or irritable, or shows somatic symptoms such as headaches. Sometimes it is manic defenses that take center stage, with behavioral disorders that can also be found in adolescents, in addition to addictions, psychotic manifestations and suicidal behavior, about which I have had the opportunity to learn a great deal while working in the adolescent crisis unit of Prof. François Ladame in Geneva.

Psychoanalysis is both a theory of psychic functioning and a method of treatment. In psychoanalytical theories, we often find the idea that the child's first "mirror" is his mother, with formulations such as "the child is reflected in his mother's gaze" or even *that he exists* through his mother's gaze – I would like to insist here in passing on the idea that it is rather a question of the primary object, as much the mother as the father. The insights of psychoanalytic theory are sometimes confirmed by modern research on the child itself, and it can now be said that the presence, absence, affect and representations that influence the way parents interact with their child play a crucial role in its development. Massimo Ammaniti and Vittorio Gallese (2014) for example have written an extensive review of current research in their book *The Birth of Intersubjectivity* where they link neurobiological research to psychodynamic theory. However, the development of the psyche remains a mystery because the infant does not have speech, and we are reduced to suppositions and interpretations by means of a language and a "secondarized"

DOI: 10.4324/9781003279297-11

thought that tries to translate processes obeying a logic that is sometimes called archaic and that escapes us by its very nature.

What I always find when I have to deal with a depressed patient, at whatever age, is low self-esteem, often translated as low self-image. Sometimes it hides behind the "grandiosity" displayed, often it ends up being verbalized, or acted out when it is a child whose palette of expression includes play. How many teenagers have I heard say that they think they are ugly when they look in the mirror or at their screen? In recent years I have been struck by the prevalence of this image issue – self-esteem seems to have become dependent on an image that becomes concrete, which is favored by the omnipresence of digital tools and the importance of social networks.

Depression is often related to loss, which is at best equivalent to the dislike of the object, at worst to the emptiness of non-existence, and/or persecution by a severe or even malicious object if it has not been integrated into a tutelary superego. It seems to me that the object these patients are afraid of losing, that they have a compulsion to identify with, becomes a persecuting object through its gaze. A gaze that is invited in order not to be alone becomes a gaze that pursues, that sends back a bad image of oneself, just as the image that the mirror sends back is experienced as ugly. I would like to illustrate these observations by an extensive case report in this volume.

From the psychoanalytic psychotherapy with Thea

The first time I saw Thea, she was in her latent period. I found a pretty, little redheaded girl in the waiting room, who struck me as inhibited. Her mother had brought her to me – she told me that something was wrong, she had become withdrawn and restless, she looked sad, lacked concentration and application in class. Recently, someone had broken the door of the house in their absence, and Thea had developed anxiety and couldn't sleep alone in her bed anymore. Her biological father had gone to live far away, and she had hardly any contact with him; she had been adopted by her mother's new husband.

Thea, who seemed absentminded in the waiting room, became more animated during the interview, while remaining reserved and at a distance. She easily gained confidence and I discovered a little girl who was happy to talk about herself with a good vocabulary and a good capacity for verbalization, understanding and symbolization. I had no indication that she might have some problems with her sense of reality. She suffered from separation anxiety with her mother and was afraid of the anger outbreaks by her adoptive father, whom she called Daddy. For the sake of simplicity, I will call him father in the following text. When I asked her how things were going with her mother, she said, "my mother makes me angry" and immediately corrected herself, "that's not what I meant, my mother is sometimes angry with me, but we can talk and make up". She also said: "My mother is sad because of the bad things Daddy says to her" (her parents were constantly having loud and ugly arguments). She was very worried because for the first time she was going to spend some weeks with her father alone. The mother later told me that she felt her daughter needed a space to talk. She herself felt too involved and helpless in the face of her daughter's complaints about the father.

I had hypothesized this little girl's fear as an oedipal anxiety: She seemed to have literally put on the maternal shoes instead of playing at being mum, since when she was with the father, he was often arguing with her. So she risked the wrath of an oedipal maternal object, in addition to receiving an overwhelming emotional charge from the father. Maybe she also feared unconsciously that he too would leave her.

Two weeks after, Thea told me a nightmare while we were playing at the dolls house. "I dreamt that I died, and I was sad that I couldn't see my mum anymore. We were both sad. When I was about to die, I woke up. I saw my cuddly toy and went back to sleep." During this session we talked about death anxieties. Thea was often invaded by fear that her mother would die. At school she didn't think about it, but she was very undisciplined during class. Then I saw Thea with her Dad. Before that meeting she had told me that, however frightened his outbursts made her, she categorically refused to talk about this with him during the session and didn't want me to mention it. I had expected to meet a frightening man. However, I met a disabled man in a wheelchair following a relatively recent accident that nobody had mentioned to me. He had narrowly escaped death after a long and complicated medical treatment. This father, a man who was aware of the negative effects of his outbursts, thought his daughter looked sad, but that it was normal under the circumstances. For him she was too withdrawn for fear of hurting her parents' feelings. He was convinced that his daughter was afraid of him because of her mother's influence.

The treatment lasted only a few months, to help the patient in the elaboration of her position in the parental conflict, to relieve the anguish linked to oedipal fantasies. She acted out scenes in the dolls house. This work quickly relieved her separation anxiety. Her time with her father went well, her grades at school went up, and the sessions became flat and repetitive. She asked if she could stop the sessions. She said she wanted to solve her problems with her father alone, and I understood that she experienced him as much too fragile to be able to bear her reproaching him; there seemed to be an almost traumatic conjunction between the father's narcissistic and physical fragility and her fear of her own wishes and impulses, which she experienced as too concrete and destructive. I let her go with mixed feelings.

Thea came to see me again after a few years. She was then a pretty, pre-teen girl, who developed gradually into a beautiful young woman arousing the interest of boys, whom she seemed to attract like flies, but to whom she had difficulty saying no. She was suffering from door-checking rituals, difficulty in falling asleep, fatigue, aboulia, constant worry. I told her that I understood that she was invaded by a fear of doing harm. She responded: "I am sometimes afraid that something will happen to my mother …. My mother is always angry with me, she always has something to blame me for. The other day I forgot to close the cage door, and our chinchilla ruined her favorite shawl."

Her destructiveness seemed to be represented in the form of this pet. I hypothesized that this was what she was trying to control in vain with her rituals, not being able to elaborate and contain it psychically. Her mother, whom she seemed unconsciously to be afraid of hurting, was at that time a fragile mother, sad following losses. During this interview, Thea mentioned very briefly that she sometimes had the phantasy that a friend was with her at home and listening to everything that was going on. During the sessions that followed, the link between destructiveness and this theme of closed–open, inside–out appeared more and more clearly. I noticed that the splitting had become rigid, and that Thea was under the threat of the loss of the object she had to protect from its destructiveness, but also under the threat of the destructiveness of the object. I told her about this animal inside her that seemed dangerous to her mother, and I showed her that her rituals were gestures to calm her anxiety – like an offering can calm someone who wants to calm the Gods who make the storms, when it has no effect on reality. This helped her, and gradually the rituals disappeared. Thea had no social difficulties, given her kind and reserved character. She never engaged in direct conflicts. Her aggressiveness was inhibited and her self weak to the point that she was unable to say no, lest she defended herself against anyone. Of course, she often found herself in relationships where her kindness was abused.

Most of the sessions then revolved around what was happening with her adoptive father. She would tell me how uncomfortable the relationship was, and I would hardly hear anything good about him. What she was telling me was indeed difficult to live with, and sometimes I found myself taking a stand, telling her that a father had no business behaving like that. I couldn't just treat it as fantasies and projection, while at the same time wondering about Thea's active part in it. Father and daughter seemed to be engaged in a dance where it was necessary to avoid too much erotic closeness without losing each other. The father struggled to maintain an adequate distance – it sometimes looked like he was talking to a wife rather than a daughter. The few times I saw them together I was struck by the atmosphere of ironic excitement in their interactions. I felt I was looking at a couple, not a father with his daughter.

The question of the gaze and the image

After some time Thea ended up telling me about what she smilingly called "her delusion". I then learned that since she was a child, she had been "summoning" people around her when she felt like it, something between delusion and imagination: She would say a formula, and then instantly feel as if they really were there, so that they could see or hear what was happening. She remembered that when she was first alone with her father, that is, when she saw me at the age of seven, she had "made" her mother sit there beside her in a cable car, and although she knew that this was impossible – she had felt it was real. She told me that once she had "summoned" someone with her in a room, and on the way out she had been afraid that she would lock him up and he would suffer, wondering at this strange mixture between imagination and reality in her mind, since she knew that he was not really there.

You can imagine that I blamed myself. She hadn't resolved the separation anxiety at the time of the first consultation by elaboration and psychic integration, but by a distortion of reality, and I had treated her on a neurotic level when she was not.

At the time she told me about it she was about 13, and was becoming embarrassed to do it, not because she was critical, but because there was a growing aspect of coercion. She couldn't always get these people to leave and was afraid that they would see or hear something they shouldn't. She was afraid that they would resent her for disposing of them without their consent, although she knew at the same time that they hadn't really been there. The fact that it was a strange relationship with reality did not worry her. (When this symptom finally disappeared, she regretted it a little: she said, "I tried it a few times, but it didn't feel the same …". She agreed that it was difficult to give up the omnipotence of being able to do what she wanted with people and find herself separated and alone in reality.) Until about the age of 14 the benefit of this omnipotence and magical thinking prevailed. But then it became very compulsive, she complained more and more about feeling obliged to summon people, and of course it interfered with her daily life, especially her school life: She became exhausted. She was having great difficulty at school and felt terrible about not living up to expectations. She had fits where she threw everything on the floor in her room, arguing with her mother and father. She started to have paranoid anxieties, and suicidal thoughts. Sometimes when she was talking to friends, she could hear her voice calling them names in her head, still knowing it was her thoughts. She showed a kind of indifference and in small doses we wondered together about this madness that was taking hold of her. She had difficulty accepting a low-dose neuroleptic treatment started at the age of 15, which she stopped as soon as she felt better, after ten months.

In therapy, Thea used me as a kind of trustful external expert, sometimes to bring her back to reality. Sometimes she seemed to expect me to give her an explanation of her reactions or what she was feeling. I felt both important and unconnected. Very rarely she could listen to what I showed her she was saying without hearing it. She often had a phobic attitude towards her thought content, which the following sequence shows: The interview takes place on the telephone that day (period of confinement for COVID 19). She calls me from home. She has put herself in a small room in the cellar, the only place in the house where she is less afraid of being heard.

She tells me about her patches (for some time now strange red patches have been forming on her skin). She can't stop checking her reflection in the mirror all the time. She looks for them to appear or disappear. When she is with someone, she can't help but feel that they are looking at her "horrible patches". She tells me that her father got angry at her in an unfair way. She tried to justify herself, but he got angry. She is afraid he will hear what she says on the phone. Suddenly she wants to check in the mirror whether there is a new patch on her skin. (She and her father have a skin disease.) When I suggest that she needs to check her patches so compulsively because, somehow, they would be a sign of her angry thoughts against her father, she reacts by telling me that it would be even worse if it were from inside her. In the sessions, I feel like a kind of reflecting mirror, literally and figuratively; she comes to reassure herself about herself in my eyes, while expecting me to think for her. I try to make her think, but often only get a kind of superficial adhesion.

Discussion

I think that paradoxically Thea cannot get depressed. She clings to a presence, remaining in the omnipotence of a magical thought that controls the other, rather than having a real inner space, something like the framing structure of the mother if we take A. Green's developments (Green, 1972). A colleague made me aware of an article by Cesar and Sarà Botella (2004), entitled "On the auto-erotic deficiency of the paranoid", which I would like to mention as a line of thought for the discussion we are going to have: They start from the idea that in the gap between the failure of the hallucinatory satisfaction of desire and the formation of the representation of the object, the infant appropriates the oral pleasure with his thumb instead of the breast through auto-eroticism:

> he takes with him, with his gaze turned inwards, the gaze of his mother ... All other sensations of the satisfaction experience gather around this axis. It is by reproducing oneself what the object brings that auto-eroticism represents the first conquest, the first autonomy.
>
> (p. 81, French edition)

Furthermore, they say:

> However, let us not be mistaken, this is more of a metaphor than a description. It is not so much a question of incorporating or introjecting the gaze, the eyes of the mother, at the psychic level, but of the child's capacity to reproduce, in a gathering at the sensorimotor level, what he feels while the mother is looking at him. In fact, when we speak of "looking at oneself", we mean the auto-erotic reproduction, independently of the object, of the original "being looked at".
>
> (p. 83 French editon)

This seems to be in line with what Vittorio Gallese (2001) says when he talks about mirror neurons in "The birth of intersubjectivity", insisting on the idea that it is a non-secondary process.

The failures of these developments would lead to an impossibility of separating, and so the paranoid must permanently cling to a real, external object, provided he can keep it within reach and at a distance, as Racamier (1966) says. But the great need for the object becomes unbearable – he hates it, and this hatred is projected, "I need his love" becomes "he hates me, he persecutes me" Racamier (1986).

But could we not consider that the way the child has been looked at may contribute to this hatred that he believes he sees in the eyes of others, or the ugliness it perceives in his reflection, in a sensory-motor mode? In Thea's case, the appearance of the patches seems to be the trace on the skin of the hatred in the link with the paternal object, this father who is really rejecting, denigrating and incomprehensible at times, a trace of a paternal incorporation linked to the very real destructiveness that this father shows with his daughter. I do agree with Bloch's developments (Bloch, 1989) arguing that the real experience with parents contributes to the development of paranoia and depression.

Conclusion

Melanie Klein theorized the importance of the depressive position as essential for normal human development. One could think that Thea needed some help to reach this position in order not to break with reality – bearing in mind that the depressed position is not equivalent to clinical depression. Studying this clinical material in the light of the developments of psycho-analysts like Botella and Botella and Racamier I have found some important clues to the understanding and importance of clinging to visual stimuli like selfies, which was Théa almost addicted to, and hallucinatory presence. One could also think that Théa regressed towards such archaic mechanisms confronted with the task of adolescent development in the context of the incestuous quality of the relationship with her adoptive father who clearly showed ambivalence towards his daughter. These lines of theoretical development seem to find an echo in the understandings developed by researchers on infantile development which we can but hope will allow us to understand better the influence of the reality of the relationship with the primary caregivers on the occurrence of mental illness.

References

Ammaniti, M., & Gallese, V. (2014). *The birth of intersubjectivity: Psychodynamics, neurobiology, and the self.* New York, NY: W.W. Norton.

Bloch, H. S. (1989). The common core of paranoia and depression. *Psychoanalytic Inquiry,* 9(3), 427–449.

Botella, C., & Botella, S. (2004). On the auto-erotic deficiency of the paranoiac. In: *The work of psychic figurability: Mental states without representation* (chap. 6). London: Routledge.

Gallese, V. (2001). The "shared manifold" hypothesis: From mirror neurons to empathy. *Journal of Consciousness Studies*, 8(5–7), 33–50.

Green, A. (1972). *The dead mother*. London: Routledge.

Palacios Espasa, F. P., & Dufour, R. (1995). *Diagnostic structurel chez l'enfant*. Paris: Masson Elsevier, pp. 81–99.

Racamier, P. C. (1966). Esquisse d'une clinique psychanalytique de la paranoïa. *Revue française de psychanalyse*, 30(1), 145–172.

Racamier, P. C. (1986). Entre agonie psychique, déni psychotique et perversion narcissique. *Revue française de psychanalyse*, 50(5), 1299–1309.

12 Early depressions

Loss of liveliness, withdrawal, psychosomatic issues and risk of developmental delay

Christine Anzieu-Premmereur

Winnicott saw the capacity to feel depressed as an achievement and a sign of health. He saw sadness and feelings of guilt as signs of achievement of the capacity for concern in a child who has a fully integrated sense of self with ego strength. But on the other side of the spectrum of mental health, Winnicott placed melancholia:

> The melancholics, who take responsibility for all the ills of the world, especially those which are quite obviously nothing to do with them, and at the other extreme are the truly responsible people of the world, those who accept the fact of their own hate, nastiness, cruelty, things which coexist with their capacity to love and to construct. Sometimes their sense of their own awfulness gets them down.
>
> If we look at depression in this way we can see that it is the really valuable people in the world who get depressed.
>
> (1958, pp. 51–52)

Melancholia and severe depression, then, are associated with "failures in the ego organization" when there has not been a good enough holding environment.

This chapter is about the body and the pre-verbal, pre-symbolic signs of depression and dissociative symptoms in infancy.

The work of melancholia

In "Mourning and Melancholia", Freud (1917) wrote about the work of melancholia as a difficult move to detach from the object that has been narcissistically invested. The ego has been identified with the object: as in the mourning process, melancholia is a narcissistic regression. The analytic treatment has to face this regression and identification, associated with the negation of it by the patient, when the depreciation of the self tries to hide the deep contempt for the object. This attack on the object is what psychoanalysts have to face when treating severely depressed patients.

The narcissistic cathexis of the object is associated with its idealization. This deep devaluation of the object is an attempt to make impossible this

DOI: 10.4324/9781003279297-12

idealization. The attack on the object associated with the introjection of the object makes the analyst face a deep self-devaluation that is a signal of the energy exerted to crash the object. When the work of melancholia is close to its end, self-esteem is regained, as being better than the idealized object. It was about accusing the object of having shown qualities and values that in fact were fake.

The intense hatred for the object had to be balanced by its narcissistic idealization. If there is a predisposition to melancholia, that should not only be the narcissistic investment in the object, but also a strong association with the hatred towards the object. The work of melancholia seems to be trying to transform this narcissistic investment in the object to make it "detachable", and the first step to take is to bind the hatred that has been the cause of the melancholic access: a binding with Eros that finally leads to sadism. The risk, if that fails, would be the depletion of the narcissistic libido that makes the patient so devaluated and guilty that suicide would be the ultimate choice.

Success in the work of melancholia seems to rely on the transformation of sadism to a masochistic capability that associates destructiveness with libidinal investments.

I would add the assumption of the role of epigenetics in the origins of depression, if we think of the postpartum time when a mother shared her mood issues with her son, while interacting closely with her infant's emotions, needs and body. This is the same for a lonely child facing absence or the frightening presence of anxious parents. It is very important to stress the role of the quality of the presence of the object, and not only the breakdown when absence becomes traumatic. The identification with parental objects that are frightening and enigmatic is associated with fear, hatred and devaluation in the ego of the patient. While a fragile narcissistic withdrawn mother can be a big source of disappointment, her idealization helps to maintain protection against the absurd non-sense of the patient's own life.

A depressed but narcissistic mother figure could be mentally absent as a "dead mother" (Green 2018), and I would like to add the specificity of a poor maternal function depleted by depression: the mother is not receptive. This lack of receiving the child's affects and absence of mirroring has created the depreciation of the self that hides the contempt for the object.

The melancholic patient cannot imagine meeting with an object that can identify with him, that could receive, accept and feel what he feels, and eventually could transform his confused negative experience. In analysis, the depressed patient can meet with an available object, interested and receptive, certainly suffering dramatically in the countertransference, but always present and available. But he resists the seduction of this new quality of sensitive accessibility.

The persecuting fantasy of being intruded by the analyst's words sometimes plays a role in the rigidity of the patient's body and his avoidance at listening to or commenting on the analyst's interpretations. Some fantasies can show pregenital sadism; for example, when being touched was unbearable. Thinking of the role of the skin ego (Anzieu, 1985), we can observe the lack of common skin with the mother and the lack of common space to think. Being touched is a source of paranoid fears and sadistic representations. The sound of the analyst's voice and the penetration in the ears could sometimes be a source of regression to a masochistic capability, with the hope of more erotic cathexis and less destructivity.

Freud (1924) pointed out how the rhythm of mother–child exchanges was a source of masochistic investment in refraining the drive discharge. This new adjustment can be seen as the binding between libidinal and destructive tensions, with more integration.

Maintaining the analytic process is a challenge facing a patient's negativity and the decathexis experienced in the countertransference.

The rhythm of the repeated sessions and the consistency of the setting help to maintain a continuous holding that hadn't been found in the early maternal presence. Fear of the patient's breakdown and suicide can punctuate the analyst's experience.

As Winnicott (1974) has shown, that fear is about a disorganization that has not been felt because of the too primitive self facing the trauma. It was repeated and fully experienced in the analysis, with primitive agonies. Those unthinkable anxieties, as Winnicott wrote, are bodily events: going to pieces, falling forever, having no orientation, and having no relationship to the body.

The blank depression in the mother and her psychic absence with which the patient as a child identified was the cause of an absence of representation: a void that doesn't allow for libidinal cathexis of a present object.

This lack of representation is what causes states of dissociation, when a melancholic patient regresses to nonverbal body impulses, like acting the infantile terror in bodily disorganization. This is when the primitive helplessness and depressive loneliness is reexperienced in the presence of the analyst, while being dissociated (Anzieu-Premmereur, 2013).

The analyst, using words to report this non-conscious traumatic event, could make the patient regain a sense of self, in a different process in the transformation of the depression.

The object and the body parts investing that presence have been annihilated in the psychotic depression. Renewing them in session with body sensations and action could be interpreted as the construction in progress of a body ego, where muscular tonus, affects and introjection of the object are associated. In some analytic sessions, the muscular activity signals how the destructivity can be discharged by motor activity and can be transformed into aggression, allowing for new energy.

That shows how regaining libidinal capacities has to do with the reintegration of a body ego in masochistic fantasies.

The patient, who cannot express with words the neglects or failures of the early environment, will signify the defect and its consequences through the body. By echoing the patient's archaic experiences, the analyst provides a circular relationship in which the perceptions and sensations are shared, contained and expressed through words.

Primary depression in babies

What is important to assess in babies is the relationship between their liveliness, their tonus of life, and the moments of disorganization–dissociation that can be understand like "anti-life" active moments. This evaluation only makes sense in relation to the characteristics of the maternal and paternal containment and shield when the father is present and willing to play his role.

A great distinction must be drawn from the outset: we have to differentiate between a picture of slump or sluggishness present very early in some babies, a state where the tonus of life would be weak from the outset, with a clinical presentation evoking an anaclitic depression as originally described by Spitz and Wolf (1946), which occurs after establishing a good relationship with the mother. The babies who have forged a real relationship with their mother are the only ones likely to react with anaclitic depression when suddenly separated from her. Babies who have failed to invest their privileged object will be indifferent to its loss.

As Palacio Espasa (2002) wrote, experiences of loss are expressed by means of three types of fantasy: catastrophic destruction of the object, the death or serious harm of the object, or rejection and loss of love of the object. Which fantasy predominates will depend on the subject's type of functioning. He described different levels of severity of depressive conflict depending, on the one hand, on the predominance of one or other fantasy expressing the loss of the object of libidinal attachment and, on the other, on the quality and intensity of the affects experienced by the ego. The affects will mobilize different defense mechanisms used by the ego, which will determine the type of psychic functioning at work.

The work on psychotic features requires a great deal of concentration on the part of the analyst, who must mobilize disorganizing components that are linked to the archaic sensory level. The pre-representational state in non-organized patients, babies as well as adults, is experienced as primarily sensorial under the dominance of primitive emotional phenomena, where analytic work helps for body recognition, awareness of living inside a body.

Analysts experience the same disconcertment when they have in the room a disorganized mother and a screaming baby who is losing her body organization: her head falling down, her limbs agitated in chaotic movements, giving the sense of a disconnection from the body. Some autistic children give the same impression of being lost and of experiencing sensorial vertigo under the pressure of unbearable sensations (Anzieu-Premmereur, 2013).

Looking at the real body and its appearance in sessions facilitates the process of revitalization in dissociated patients.

The body is the point of origin of the ego, wrote Freud. In treating difficult patients, we confront explosive disorganization, uncontainable acting out, or de-emotionalized states, with patients who are deprived of life, who have no "texture", and who remain estranged from symbolic functioning.

The sense of a lack of "being" when the self is damaged by frustration – whether because the baby has a very low level of tolerance or because the environment fails to provide the necessary support – militates against the process of creating representations. Babies who have had avoidant reactions to their mother suffer as toddlers from disorganizing separation anxieties. In their confusion, they experience the mother being absent forever. There is no memory that could keep her alive.

Autoerotism, with its infinite potential for playing out the recreation of memories, helps to associate sensations and representations and to develop further displacements. Autoerotism is for the subject a background on which the imago is represented. Infantile sexuality starts out from there.

The affect associated with the process can change the perception, since the psyche can transform, deny or neglect the external reality. The roots of the representational capacity are fully linked with the affect. In cases of early trauma, violent affects will be discharged and destabilize the psyche and its ability for representation and symbolization.

Early defenses such as splitting, denial, decathexis or expulsion of the psyche outside of the body, somatic reactions and foreclosure will then interfere with any representational process.

As Bowlby (1960) and Winnicott (1948) each in their own way have pointed out, it's not the separation that causes the baby to suffer depression, it's the loss of hope. An object that has disappeared as much as it is inaccessible, for example during an abrupt weaning from the breast, or interacting with an inanimate mother without vocalization or staring, or an illness, a surgical intervention, all these can remove the links with the object. The infant is sluggish, withdrawn, slowed down, rapidly psychosomatically disorganized, and may present the pathological defenses described by Selma Fraiberg (1982): avoidance of eye contact, paralysis of behavior or freezing, transformation of affects when, instead of manifesting distress or anguish, an abused baby manifests loud joy and disorganized excitement and self-aggression.

In the perinatal period, between 0 and 6 months, reactions which are called depressive in the small baby are rather reactions of collapse of the tone of life, loss of the possibility of investing, than reactions to the loss of an object which in fact is not yet solidly constituted. We observe infants with blank expressions, not smiling, no joyful expression in the eyes, but rather indifferent, rarely surprised; they look away, vocalize very little, with slow gestures and lack of postural anticipation when being hugged. These babies have lost their skills, and are detached from others as from themselves.

At the beginning of life, the body is still fragile, and maintaining the sensations and experience of being alive through movements, through the action of the body is essential. Restoring bodily dialogue is urgent. It is the economic aspect of maternal psychic functioning that is communicated to the child in the dance of pre-verbal games. Prosody, the rhythm of the utterance as well as of the porterage, the intensity of the gaze and of the voice are essential signals to which the baby responds with its own register of primitive drive.

In analytic interventions, the triangulation associated with the presence of the therapist in front of the mother–infant dyad, or the mobilization of the paternal presence at the insistent invitation of the analyst, modifies the libidinal investment of the baby for a "Non-mother" character who has an essential anti-depressive impact by modifying the constellation of anxieties and defenses which characterizes the little child when he reaches the depressive position. This new connection allows for a bridge between the analyst and the baby.

The great models of play are organized around absence: fort da, hide and seek are games of controlled loss. The discovery and creation of games, pleasures of all registers, the re-sexualization of life, always show an improvement in a baby; the appearance of smiles in impassive infants, of laughter in infants who have finally become enthusiastic, are reliable signs of change. Joint therapies provide support for both mother and child to deal with each other's damaged narcissism; toddler's depressive collapses are always attacks on the integrity of the self that can have serious developmental consequences.

This is why it is essential to intervene quickly and early when we see worrying signs in babies, but it is still difficult to know the long-term influence of these interventions. The consequences of primary collapses are multiple throughout life, from early childhood disorders, such as developmental delays or attention difficulties, to serious obstacles to access to oedipal conflict, damage to adolescence and traumatic repetitions in adulthood.

Even if they regain their vital capacity with therapy, some young children will develop a problem of motor and behavioral discharge bypassing the transitional issues that are essential to underpin the thickness of preconscious functioning and would allow a thinking activity to develop.

A five-month-old detached baby

When I met Tom, he was a floppy five-month-old baby in the arms of a borderline distressed mother. He was listless, anorectic, showed no interest in the surrounding world; motionless, insensitive, always calm, showing no spontaneous emotion. He seemed to take no pleasure in anything, with no curiosity for others. His mother was sobbing. They spent entire days in bed, she watching television, crying, whilst he was sucking his mother's hair. The baby did not fill up the void in her and sought to compensate for the lack of relationship in self-stimulation.

During the night, Tom was sleepless, scratching his skin, while during the day, he had outbursts of disorganizing rage.

We had been meeting for several months and 14-month-old Tom knew me well. He arrived covered with bruises and his mother explained that he was really stupid because he repeatedly fell off his chair. Tom immediately climbed onto a stool and dropped down. I told him that he had been afraid of falling down for a long time when he was an infant, and that he had felt lost. He looked at me attentively and started again, but without hurting himself. His mother rushed over to him. I told them that when mommy cried, Tom felt like she let him down. Tom took a toy he found in his mother's bag and threw it at me; we played swap and I included the mother in the game, but she wouldn't join in the game and found it all silly.

But Tom needed to repeat the game; he was adept at catching up with the object that belonged to both him and his mother. He started to jump on the couch, finding a certain tone for the first time, and letting himself fall violently into the arms of his mother who welcomed him for once. This game of falling and knocking then became a ritual in the sessions. Tom had regained his vitality and his weight curve improved; and even if his mother still found our games "silly", she participated in them.

Tom created a play when he pretended to feed me, removing the spoon as soon as I leaned towards him. He laughed at my frustration and his sadistic control of the situation. I said to him: "You are making me a good joke!" His mother was surprised, she had never heard him laugh.

Tom had been an anorexic baby since a brutal withdrawal when he was four months old had left him sluggish, lacking in energy, collapsed.

Active in this new game, Tom was then able to become passive again in the face of his mother playing at devouring him, becoming an object of desire for her, thus restoring part of his wounded narcissism and regaining a new libidinal quality.

When he was four, Tom told me how distressed he was when being forced to take a bath since he felt his body melting in the water like powdered sugar. He compulsively drew animals with multiple skins, the sign of a double skin formation that babies build when their narcissistic early support has been too "thin". The fantasy of a common skin with the mother should have helped to figure out a container of psychic experience, described as essential for maintaining a capacity for internal organization.

As in Ferenczi's (1929) description of destructiveness in "unwelcome" children, psychoanalysts observing infants have emphasized the impact of primary body rejection on negativity and violence in childhood.

Many non-neurotic patients have been confronted very early on with issues regarding the penetrability of their primal environment: the spontaneous maternal capacity to sustain sufficient passivation to allow the infant's projective identification without having to make excessive effort to penetrate the object. Like Patrick Miller presented recently, the quality of penetrability is both psychic and bodily (Miller, 2014).

Patients come to analysis with the unconscious wish that they will find the capacity to experience normal projective identification, with the soma-topsychic interpenetration that it allows and that stimulates psychic growth.

This requires what we know from Ferenczi – a bisexual capacity in the analyst to be penetrable and actively passive.

Conclusion

The topic of melancholic depression addresses the question of the emergence of early forms of symbol representation that are produced within the mode of presence of the object. Those processes are anchored in sensory–motricity.

Failures in early encounters with the maternal object are followed by an affect of "primary narcissistic disappointment" and mobilize a procession of primitive defense mechanisms (Fraiberg, 1982) in which, at one end we see the early forms of retreat in an autistic line and at the other, the attempts at healing by an intensified masochism (Roussillon 2018).

Since Freud noted that the object choice of the melancholic is narcissistic, everyone agrees that depressed patients expect from their object not only satisfaction of desire, but something which seems essentially narcissistic. The depressed patient is anxious about keeping a common link with his object, which is idealized, and of which, at the same time, the otherness cannot support: the object has only a functional value.

It seems to me that melancholic patients in analysis can regain some vitality by recovering a masochistic capability that is less damaging than it seems. This is more the signal of the recovery of a libidinal cathexis and identification, than one of an aggrieving pathology. The severe melancholic pain can then shift to a feeling of guilt – but no shame anymore – and hurting oneself, in actions closely associated with primitive bodily anxieties that were finally shared with the containing analyst (Reith et al., 2018).

The remarkable adaptability of the analyst plays the role of the holding environment, and his creativity, while suffering the negativeness and hatred of the damaged patient, can help to accomplish the challenge to transform melancholic pain and deadly impulses into ambivalent feelings in a lively body ego.

References

Anzieu, D. (1985). *The skin ego* (new translation). London: Karnac2016.

Anzieu-Premmereur, C. (2013). The process of representation in early childhood. In: H. Levine, G. Reed & D. Scarfone (Eds.), *The work of figurability: From unrepresented to represented mental states* (pp. 240–254). London: Routledge.

Bowlby, J. (1960). Grief and mourning in infancy and early childhood. *The Psychoanalytic Study of the Child*, 15(1), 9–52.

Ferenczi, S. (1929). The unwelcome child and his death-instinct. *International Journal of Psycho-Analysis*, 10, 125–129.

Freud, S. (1917). Mourning and melancholia, *S.E.* 14.

Freud, S. (1924). The economic problem of masochism, *S.E.* 19.

Fraiberg, S. (1982). Pathological defenses in infancy. *The Psychoanalytic Quarterly*, 51(4), 612–635.

Green, A. (2018). The dead mother complex. In: *Parent–infant psychodynamics* (pp. 162–174). London: Routledge.

Miller, P. (2014). *Driving soma: A transformational process in the analytic encounter*. London: Karnac.

Palacio Espasa, F. (2002). Considerations on depressive conflict and its different levels of intensity: Implications for technique. *The International Journal of Psychoanalysis*, 83(4), 825–836.

Reith, B., Moller, M., Boots, J., Crick, P., Gibeault, A., Jaffe, R., ... & Vermote, R. (2018). Countertransference and enactment. In: B. Reith, M. Møller, J. Boots, P.

Crick, A. Gibeault, R. Jaffè, ... & R. Vermote (2018). *Beginning analysis: On the processes of initiating psychoanalysis.* London: Routledge.

Roussillon, R. (2018). *Primitive agony and symbolization.* New York: Routledge.

Spitz, R. A., & Wolf, K. M. (1946). Anaclitic depression: An inquiry into the genesis of psychiatric conditions in early childhood, II. *The psychoanalytic study of the child*, 2(1), 313–342.

Winnicott, D. W. (1948). Reparation in respect of mother's organized defense against depression. In: *1958 Collected Papers: Through Pediatrics to Psycho-Analysis.* London: Tavistock.

Winnicott, D. W. (1958). The family affected by depressive illness in one or both parents. In: *The family and individual development.* London: Tavistock.

Winnicott, D. W. (1974). Fear of breakdown. *International Review of Psychoanalysis,* 1: 103–107.

13 Pluralism in psychoanalytic research

Conceptual framework of the MODE study

Gilles Ambresin, Tamara Fischmann and Marianne Leuzinger-Bohleber

Research in psychoanalysis has developed by focusing primarily on the patient–analyst encounter, resulting in clinical–psychoanalytic research as well as conceptual research. Developed by Freud in a close interconnection between the brain and the psyche (Freud, 2006[1895]) as well as in the scientific context of his time (Makari, 2008), psychoanalysis was conceived from the beginning as a plural science of the unconscious (Leuzinger-Bohleber. 2018). Thus, contemporary so-called extra-clinical psychoanalytic research sets out to explore the complexity of the analytic encounter through plural and relevant scientific perspectives considering the understanding that the gap between the clinical encounter and the requirements of the scientific–empirical approach cannot be bridged by a single heuristic method (Steinmair & Löffler-Stastka, 2021). Finally, although the effectiveness of psychoanalytic therapy for various disorders has been demonstrated (Leichsenring & Klein, 2020), research findings contribute little to clinical practice (Shedler, 2010). Work to close this gap between psychoanalytic research and clinical practice is needed (Shedler, 2010). The purpose of this chapter is to address the aforementioned issues in analytic therapy research with the belief that sharing findings, methods, and questions about empirical research supports the development of clinical skills and critical thinking for both students and senior analytic therapy clinicians. In an attempt to achieve these goals, the chapter will first discuss the conceptual framework of psychoanalytic research, followed by an example of research and a conclusion that psychoanalytic studies emanating from plural sources are necessary and complementary for the advancement of the science of the unconscious.

Conceptual framework

The conceptual framework of psychoanalytic research was from its inception placed within a perspective of a plural science of the unconscious (Leuzinger-Bohleber, 2018). Freud's formative journey provides insight into how psychoanalysis brings together plural sources and has done so from its conception.

DOI: 10.4324/9781003279297-13

Reminder of Freud's background

Freud defined psychoanalysis as "the science of the unconscious", which may have seemed like an oxymoron to some. During his medical training, he worked for six years in neurological research in Ernst Brücke's laboratory, where he was confronted with a strictly positivist conception of science that would accompany him throughout his life. Freud later turned away from the neurology of his time, recognizing the methodological limits of this discipline for the investigation of the psyche. In embarking on this research, Freud integrated ideas and scientific evidence from many fields of his time to form a new discipline: "the goal was to win for science the traditional object of humanist culture, the inner life of human beings" (Makari, 2008, 3). This attempt was not without resistance in the medical world, with Freud commenting on the reception of the communication of his neurotic findings to the Association for Psychiatry and Neurology as follows, "I was annoyed by the very reduced understanding I found there; I withdrew again" (Makari, 2008). It was during this same year that Freud wrote a *Psychology for Neurologists* which was never published during his lifetime and is better known as the *Project for a Scientific Psychology*. For the purpose of this article, it is interesting to note that the qualifier "scientific" was given by Strachey, whereas Freud may have spoken of a "first sketch of psychology" (Freud, 2006[1895], 180). The intention of the *Project* was to provide a psychology pertaining to the natural sciences (Freud, 2006[1895], 603). The possibilities of a neurophysiological or strictly psychoanalytical reading of this text have been debated, but what is certain is that the years that follow Freud's thinking will broaden its scope. And rather than speaking of a transition from a neurophysiological model to a psychological referential, we could speak of a new stratum of Freud's thought, which allows us to consider psychoanalysis as a plural science of the unconscious. The sedimentation of this new stratum carried out by Freud can be illustrated by the intellectual work around the *Project of a Psychology* which dates from 1895 and the *Interpretation of the Dreams*, essentially completed in 1896, but in 1899 for Chapter VII. In Chapter VII, Freud states that he will remain on the psychological terrain (Freud, 2003 [1900a], 589). A "goodbye" but not a farewell, for the scientific positivism of his beginnings would continue to guide Freud and he would never completely give up on his project. Freud did not reach the destination he had hoped for in his 1897 letter to Fliess during his lifetime. It is only at the very end of the 20th century that a strong questioning of the place of biology in psychotherapy (Kandel, 1998) and in particular in psychoanalysis (Kandel, 1999) re-emerged. While waiting for more precise exploration reserved for those who will come after him (Freud, 2006[1897]), Freud engaged in the exploration of the human psyche which, to be scientifically knowable, must be, and Freud insists, established by laws, deterministic and not based on random events (Makari, 2008, 77). Freud was thus interested in experimental studies that would allow him to support his new psychology. Freud wrote to Jung:

Now that you, Bleuler and to some extent Löwenfeld have won me a hearing among the readers of scientific literature ... the movement in favour of our new ideas will continue irresistibly despite all the efforts of the moribund authorities.

(Makari, 2008, 197)

Psychoanalysts after Freud will continue their research efforts on these foundations of plural science of the unconscious. After these historical elements that have shown the plurality of references in the construction of psychoanalysis, we can present a global conceptual scheme to better understand the richness of research in psychoanalysis today.

Overall conceptual scheme

At the center of psychoanalytic research stands the analytic session. With it and around it, we can distinguish two different groups of psychoanalytic research – the group of clinical research and the group of extra-clinical research. Clinical research is comprised of psychoanalytic research in the psychoanalytic situation itself as well as of conceptual research. Extra-clinical research takes place after the psychoanalytic sessions and encompasses a variety of research strategies.

Clinical research (clinical–psychoanalytical)

Clinical research takes place in the intimacy of the psychoanalytical situation. It puts at work the psychic apparatuses of the analyst and the analysand. We will concentrate on the analyst. The psychoanalytic situation can be described as the meeting of the analytic site and the analyzing situation (Donnet, 2005, 19–21). The analyzing situation characterizes: "the specific functional unit comprised of the set analysand–analyst situation: the unit of connection between the patient's intrapsychic processes and their externalisation on the transference scene" (Donnet, 2005, 20). The psychoanalytic situation can be represented as a circular process of discovery (Figure 13.1) within this functional unit by which idiosyncratic observations of unconscious fantasies and conflicts are successively visualized, symbolized and finally put into words in "metapsychological snapshots" (Rolland, 2020). This activity seeks to make the experience of the encounter and the clinical observation speakable and transmissible. Only a small part of these is accessible to the analyst's conscious thinking. This understanding inevitably shapes the processes of perception of subsequent clinical situations, both in the same treatment and in other treatments. In the daily clinical practice, psychoanalytic research is thus oriented towards the exploration of the appearances of the unconscious in its clinical manifestations in order to try to draw out the laws that govern them in this individual during a given session, but also towards the possible extraction, at a more or less distant time, of laws with a more general scope, beyond the

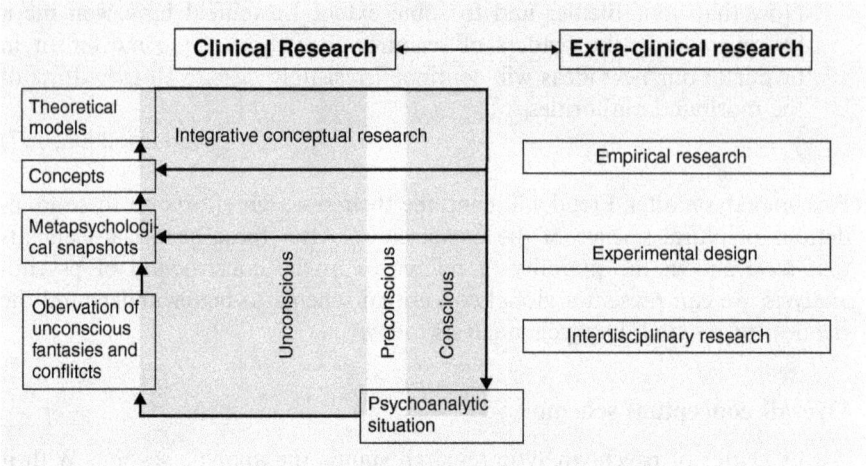

Figure 13.1 Psychoanalytic research: a plural science of the unconscious (adapted from Leuzinger-Bohleber, 2015b, 21).

session. The psychoanalytic process of research in session is carried out by trial and error and results in the emergence of "unconscious truths" that take the place of evidence. Its outcome always remains open and perfectible (Alfandary, 2021), so it can be characterized as a critical hermeneutic.

Conceptual research

Clear psychoanalytic concepts can help to advance the establishment of an acceptable methodology for third party review of results. Conceptual research is one of many other forms of psychoanalytic research and aims to clarify psychoanalytic concepts. The development of psychoanalysis as a science and as a clinical practice has always depended heavily on various forms of conceptual research. Conceptual research has clarified, formulated, and reformulated psychoanalytic concepts to better shape the outcomes emerging in the clinical setting.

Concepts emerge from the psychological and research work of the functional unit of analyst–analyst situation, as well as from the work of secondarization that takes place in the supervisions (Figure 13.1). New loops are drawn with "feedback" both on the psychoanalytic situation and on metapsychological snapshots and concepts, thus drawing an integrative conceptual research activity.

By decreasing the elasticity of concepts, improving the clarity and explicitness of concept use, conceptual research has facilitated the integration of existing psychoanalytic thinking as well as the development of new ways of looking at clinical and extra-clinical data.

In addition, it has offered conceptual bridges to neighboring disciplines particularly interested in psychoanalysis.

Extra-clinical research

On the basis of the results of clinical and conceptual psychoanalytic research, extra-clinical research in psychoanalysis can develop. It investigates the results of this research with its own means of investigation. Extra-clinical research can make use of empirical, experimental and interdisciplinary studies.

By *empirical research* we mean studies that are based on observations and measurable facts. The place of empirical research has been, and may still be, controversial in the psychoanalytic community. So much so that, "Empirical, and especially quantitative research in psychoanalysis and the dialogue with the natural sciences were considered by many as naive and unsuited to psychoanalysis, even to the point of being harmful" (Leuzinger-Bohleber, 2015b, 19). It must be acknowledged that it can be difficult for the trained psychoanalyst, steeped in clinical experience, to meet the demands of scientists and academics trained in demanding methodologies. To imagine the clinical practice of psychoanalysis and its constraints is certainly also difficult for extra-clinical researchers. Moreover, careful extra-clinical research always requires a great deal of effort, which can only be provided by a network of well-equipped researchers, committed clinicians, and constant reflection on the interdependencies of each other's heuristic models. However, the gap between the two positions seems to be narrowing, as shown for example by the publication of the book *Neuroscience and Psychoanalysis* (Magistretti & Ansermet, 2010).

Experimental research uses methods outside the psychoanalytic field such as magnetic resonance imaging (MRI) or electroencephalogram (EEG) to undertake an experimental exploration of particular psychoanalytic concepts, such as dreams.

Interdisciplinary research builds bridges with other research fields. Examples such as the links with attachment research, developmental empirical research, but also literature or cultural studies, show the creativity of these exchanges. These three categories can be combined.

Multimodal neuroimaging outcome study of psychoanalytic psychotherapy in with chronic depression (MODE)

The example of MODE is intended to illustrate the challenges of extra-clinical research in psychoanalytic treatment. MODE asks the following question: "Do successful psychotherapies lead to changes in the structures and functions of the brain?" Studies on this question are still rare, but of great importance for contemporary psychoanalytic research, as they may discover neurobiological mechanisms that are crucial for lasting changes, particularly in severely mentally ill patients. Patients with chronic depression (CD) belongs to this group of patients and CD is still difficult to treat nowadays. At the time the idea for MODE emerged, clinical practice guidelines for CD recommended the provision of a psychotherapeutic treatment that addresses their specific needs and deficits (Jobst et al., 2016).

The outcomes of long-term psychoanalytic psychotherapy with CD were highlighted in the LAC study (Leuzinger-Bohleber et al., 2019a, 2019b). The LAC study compared the effectiveness of long-term cognitive-behavioral therapy (CBT) and long-term psychoanalytic therapy (PAT) in 252 chronically depressed patients (Beutel et al., 2012). Both psychotherapies showed a clinically relevant and highly significant reduction of depressive symptoms over 1, 2, and 3 years. After 3 years, self-rated full remission rates were 45% (BDI $\leq$ 12) and clinician-rated full remission rates were 61% (QIDS-C $\leq$ 5). The effect sizes were very large, d = 1.78 (BDI), and d = 2.12 (QIDS-C). As in other studies, the researchers found no significant differences between PAT and CBT concerning symptom reduction (Leuzinger-Bohleber et al., 2019a). However, they achieved better effect sizes and full remission rates compared to other studies (see e.g., Steinert et al. 2014). Three years after the start of treatment, significantly more patients in PAT showed structural changes compared to patients in CBT (Leuzinger-Bohleber et al., 2019b).

An unexpected finding of the LAC study was that PAT led to good, even sustaining, structural transformation as well as to changes in symptom severity in CD patients with childhood maltreatment (CM), especially if they received therapy at a high weekly frequency. Hence, MODE will compare the effects of low-frequency (LF) vs high-frequency (HF) PAT.

Clinical research development of a manual for a disorder specific psychoanalytic intervention

This first phase of the development of a psychoanalytic intervention that addresses the specificities of CD requires clinical psychoanalytic thinking. In psychoanalytic long-term treatment, the focus of therapeutic change is on the transformation of the patient's unconscious mental world, the self- and object-representations as well as unresolved developmental conflicts that influence thinking, acting, and feeling and lead to maladaptation to the patients' present environment. Psychoanalytic literature has therefore emphasized again and again the importance of change in mental structures and not only symptoms for a sustained transformation of the patients' emotional functioning. To achieve such structural change is still regarded as one of the unique features of psychoanalysis. As regards MODE, however, such general objectives should meet the specific objectives of addressing CD and CM. Hence, the manual devotes a section to the general tasks and basic psychoanalytic attitudes in the treatment of patients with CD and CM as well as a section on the specific tasks in treating them. Manual use may induce the concern to psychoanalysts that general psychoanalytic attitudes and aims will be constrained (Kächele, 2013; Shedler, 2018). The MODE manual does not provide a "cookbook" approach to treatment but rather acknowledges and emphasizes that the group of patients with CD and CM requires a great deal of creativity, originality, and flexibility in the psychoanalyst's treatment technique in order to be able to reach the patient emotionally at all (Leuzinger-

Bohleber, Fischmann, & Beutel, 2021). In sum, The MODE manual intends to provide suggestions for the psychoanalytic treatment of these difficult-to-treat patients while respecting the general principles of psychoanalysis.

Extra-clinical research manual development

While this first stage has essentially clinical and conceptual psychoanalytic research aspects, it also has an extra-clinical research aspect. Indeed, the manual will serve as a reference base for clinicians during treatment as well as for clinical discussions in the framework of supervisions. In extra-clinical research, it is important to establish that the treatment delivered is consistent with that prescribed by the study. The manual, by establishing key concepts, helps to verify that therapists are providing treatment consistent with MODE. Adherence to treatment is established by external judges, which requires recording a number of sessions. Therapists may be reluctant to accept the recording of sessions. Some may argue that it intrudes on the privacy of the analytic session. Our experience shows that these are initial fears of clinicians, and the recorder is quickly forgotten. Few patients object to it. However, good communication with clinicians is important.

Extra-clinical research development of the research protocol

To be accepted in the medical field, a new treatment must demonstrate its effectiveness according to the principles of evidence-based medical research. To meet this requirement, a research protocol corresponding to the gold standard of medical research, the randomized controlled trial, was developed. In MODE, adult patients (21–60 years) are recruited and included in the study if they present with CD (duration >2 years) of a certain severity and CM (at least one trauma on the Childhood Trauma Questionnaire subscales). They are then randomly assigned to LF or HF PAT.

A challenge for the linkage between clinical practice and extra-clinical research appears here since patients are allocated to treatment according to inclusion criteria and not to clinical indication. Studies show contrasting results with regard to the effect of randomization. A recent meta-analysis showed that receiving a preferred treatment was moderately and positively associated with the rate of treatment discontinuation and the therapeutic alliance. However, the authors did not find a significant association with clinical outcomes (Windle et al., 2020). A previous meta-analysis showed that patient preferences modestly but consistently affected treatment satisfaction and completion as well as clinical outcomes (Lindhiem et al., 2014). In the LAC study, receiving the preferred treatment did not provide better clinical outcomes than in the group of patients randomly assigned to treatment. However, in the authors' opinion, patients were clearly reluctant to randomize (Leuzinger-Bohleber et al., 2019a). In summary, the effect of randomization on clinical outcomes remains an open question.

Extra-clinical research: the example of neuroscience

In a recent study, Bansal and colleagues (2018) yoked multi-modal MRI to a 10-week randomized, placebo-controlled trial of an antidepressant medication in treating unmedicated adults with Persistent Depressive Disorder. They acquired 121 anatomical MRI scans in 41 depressed patients before the start and at the end of the trial, and once in 29 matched healthy controls. At study baseline, the depressed group had significantly thicker cortices than the controls, and in inverse proportion to the severity of depressive symptoms, suggesting that hypertrophy was adaptive and helped to attenuate symptoms. Medication reduced symptoms compared with placebo, and it normalized cortical thickness (CT) measures, whereas placebo had no effect. Mediation analyses showed that medication reduced CT through the reduction of symptoms (rather than reducing symptoms by way of normalizing CT); these findings suggested that adaptive cortical plasticity was no longer needed in those who responded to medication, and therefore thickness values returned to normal with successful treatment. This study demonstrated the importance of neural plasticity of the cortical mantle in mediating the effects of treatment on attenuating depressive symptoms. Following on from those findings, MODE will examine the effects of PAT on CT as the primary outcome, while psychological measures will also be collected. Overall objectives in MODE are to investigate whether and how the brain structure, function, and metabolism of CD patients with CM will change after one year of manualized PAT. More specifically, MODE will investigate whether and how CD patients with CM receiving 1- or 3-weekly session PAT show differential changes in MRI-based brain measures, from baseline to 1 year and how brain measures are associated with clinical therapeutic achievements.

Thanks to evidence gathered throughout the study, MODE could contribute clinically to grant CD patients with CM access to a treatment that addresses their specific needs. From a research perspective, were MODE to demonstrate successfully convergent multimodal changes, this would be an important step forward to open significant perspectives for integrative and translational research. This field of research will enrich mutual understanding of discipline-specific mechanisms of change. Despite those perspectives and while brain changes and changes in psychological measures such as severity of depression are recognized indicators of change in the scientific community, these measures report changes at the group level (e.g. means). Psychoanalysts, both clinicians and researchers, are also interested in changes in psychological structure as well as in changes at the individual level.

Changes in psychoanalytic measures dreams and neuroscience

One way to address this issue is to focus on a well-known psychoanalytic concept, dreams. Dreams are still considered to be one of the "via regiae" to the patient's unconscious in contemporary psychoanalysis. Changes in manifest dreams as well as transformations in latent dream contents approached in psychoanalytical sessions are plausible clinical indicators for psychoanalysts that the unconscious world of inner objects and associated fantasies and conflicts might have been modified. Support for the assertion that dreams are meaningful indicators of mental functioning is found in a review article summarizing the results of recent sleep dream research (Siclari, Valli & Arnulf, 2020): "Importantly, these studies convincingly show that dream reports can be trusted as a research tool, and that they do not represent confabulations or unreliable indications, as has often been suggested" (p. 856). Authors emphasize that the new neuroimaging techniques (EEG, MRI, fMRI, PET and high-density EEG) have opened up promising perspectives for research in this field. This perspective was considered in the Frankfurt EEG/Depression study (FRED study), which investigated dreams in a sub-sample of patients in the LAC study by using neuroscientific methods (fMRI, EEG). Authors were able to demonstrate systematic neurobiological changes recalling a significant dream after one and a half years of psychoanalytic treatment compared with the remembering processes of the same dream at the beginning of treatment (Fischmann, Russ & Leuzinger-Bohleber, 2013).

Overall, findings gained with the help of neuroscience are consistent with previous clinical–psychoanalytical research and provide further indications of changes in dreams as a mechanism of change in psychoanalysis.

Empirical research informs clinical technique

In MODE, dream diaries will be collected and analyzed using a coding system with formal criteria (Moser & von Zeppelin, 1996). Based on their model of cognitive–affect regulation, this evaluation system can be used to investigate manifest dream–content and its changing structures (Fischmann et al., 2013). Analyses of dreams in the FRED study suggested that changes in the manifest dream contents as well as in the association of the dream (indicators for the latent dream content) can thus be used as signs for often hidden transformations during psychoanalyses. For example, if the dream–subject gains a more active stance and control over a dangerous situation and is no longer exclusively a passive, lonely victim but in company with helping others often means that there are "turning points" in the psychoanalytical process. Another indicator noted by the authors is the systematic change of affects in the manifest dreams: the spectrum is enlarged. Not one single affect dominates the dream plot anymore as in the initial phase of the treatment (Leuzinger-Bohleber, 2015a).

Results of this research show the importance of changes in manifest dream–content. They indicate to the clinician that it would be beneficial for their patient to give them particular importance in treatment. Indeed, a difficulty in treating patients with severe CD is addressing psychic pain and helping them cope with the unbearable thoughts that often underlie depression (Leuzinger-Bohleber et al., 2019b). Clinicians who turn their attention to this psychic pain as featured in manifest dream–contents certainly help patients strengthen the self and regain a sense of autonomy and agentivity. Of course, these dream case studies are too isolated to formulate clinical recommendations. However, they reveal preliminary aspects that can draw clinicians' attention to these aspects in their clinical practice and support their activity as clinical "researchers" with their patients. These case studies feed conceptual psychoanalytic research and empirical research in return.

Conclusion

To summarize, this chapter has gone through the conceptual framework of psychoanalytic research which can be divided into three main areas: clinical research, conceptual research, and extra-clinical research. This journey into empirical research showed that research supports the effectiveness of psychoanalytic treatment and that it also allows therapeutic concepts closer to the clinician to be studied. It has particularly addressed the aspect of extra-clinical research based on the example of the MODE study. This study falls into several categories, since it proposes a treatment in a psychoanalytical setting, which calls for clinical and conceptual research, with an experimental design that opens up a space for extra-clinical research. By presenting MODE, this journey has sought to show how empirical research questions arise from the clinical experience and feed back into it. The development of mixed methods may support the return of the case study to an empirical context in such a way that it enriches both the research and the clinical session. Further, case study complements the positivist scientific paradigm with a constructivist perspective, which is more likely to provide knowledge emerging from practice. This allows for a wide range of data to be collected in a collaborative research effort to advance research in the science of the unconscious. Through these examples, this journey aimed to help reduce the gap too often encountered between research and clinic practice by presenting research in psychoanalysis as a plural field of inquiry into the unconscious.

References

Alfandary, I. (2021). *Science et fiction chez Freud. Quelle épistémologie pour la psychanalyse?* Paris: Éditions d'Ithaque.

Bansal, R., Hellerstein, D. J., & Peterson, B. S. (2018). Evidence for neuroplastic compensation in the cerebral cortex of persons with depressive illness. *Molecular Psychiatry*, 23(2), 375–383.

Beutel, M., Leuzinger-Bohleber, M., Rüger, B., Bahrke, U., Negele, A., Haselbacher, A. et al. (2012). Psychoanalytic and cognitive-behavior therapy of chronic depression: Study protocol for a randomized controlled trial. *Trials*, 13, 117. Available at: www.trialsjournal.com/content/pdf/1745-6215-13-117.pdf

Donnet, J. L. (2005). *La situation analysante*. Paris: Presses universitaires de France.

Fischmann, T., Russ, M. O., & Leuzinger-Bohleber, M. (2013). Trauma, dream, and psychic change in psychoanalyses: A dialog between psychoanalysis and the neurosciences. *Frontiers in Human Neuroscience*, 7. doi:10.3389/fnhum.2013.00877.

Freud, S. (2003[1900a]). *L'interprétation du rêve*, Chap. VII. *OCF* IV. Paris: PUF.
Freud, S. (2006[1895]) *Lettres à Fliess*. Paris: PUF.
Freud, S. (2006[1897]) *Lettres à Fliess*. Paris: PUF.
Jobst, A., Brakemeier, E-L., Buchheim, A., Caspar, F., Cuijpers, P., Ebmeier, K. P., Falkai, P., van der Gaag, R. J., Gaebel, W., Herpertz, S., Kurimay, T., Sabaß, L., Schnell, K., Schramm, E., Torrent, C., Wasserman, D., Wiersma, J., & Padberg, F. (2016). European Psychiatric Association guidance on psychotherapy in chronic depression across Europe. *European Psychiatry*, 33(1), 18–36.
Kächele, H. (2013). Manualization as tool in psychodynamic psychotherapy research and clinical practice: Commentary on six studies. *Psychoanalytic Inquiry*, 33(6), 626–630.
Kandel, E. R. (1998). A new intellectual framework for psychiatry. *American Journal of Psychiatry*, 155(4), 457–469.
Kandel, E. R. (1999). Biology and the future of psychoanalysis: a new intellectual framework for psychiatry revisited. *American Journal of Psychiatry*, 156(4), 505–524.
Leichsenring, F., & Klein, S. (2020). Evidence for psychodynamic psychotherapy in specific mental disorders. *Outcome research and the future of psychoanalysis: Clinicians and researchers in dialogue* (pp. 99–127). New York: Routledge.
Leuzinger-Bohleber, M. (2015a). Working with severely traumatized, chronically depressed analysands. *The International Journal of Psychoanalysis*, 96(3), 611–636.
Leuzinger-Bohleber, M. (2015b). Development of a plurality during the hundred year-old history of research of psychoanalysis. In: M. Leuzinger-Bohleber & H. Kächele (Eds.), *An open door review of outcome and process studies in psychoanalysis* (pp. 17–41). International Psychoanalytic Association. www.ipa.world/en/Psychoanalytic_Theory/Research/open_door.aspx
Leuzinger-Bohleber, M. (2018). Psychoanalysis as a "science of the unconscious" and its dialogue with the neurosciences and embodied cognitive science: Some historical and epistemological remarks. In: *Finding the body in the mind* (pp. 1–18). London: Routledge.
Leuzinger-Bohleber, M., Fischmann, T., & Beutel, M. (2021). *Analytische Langzeitpsychotherapien von chronisch depressiven Patienten (LAC Manual)*. Göttingen: Hogrefe Publishing.
Leuzinger-Bohleber, M., Hautzinger, M., Fiedler, G., Keller, W., Bahrke, U., Kallenbach, L., ... & Beutel, M. (2019a). Outcome of psychoanalytic and cognitive-behavioural long-term therapy with chronically depressed patients: a controlled trial with preferential and randomized allocation. *The Canadian Journal of Psychiatry*, 64(1), 47–58.
Leuzinger-Bohleber, M., Kaufhold, J., Kallenbach, L., Negele, A., Ernst, M., Keller, W., ... & Beutel, M. (2019b). How to measure sustained psychic transformations in long-term treatments of chronically depressed patients: Symptomatic and structural changes in the LAC Depression Study of the outcome of cognitive-behavioural and psychoanalytic long-term treatments. *The International Journal of Psychoanalysis*, 100(1), 99–127.
Lindhiem, O., Bennett, C. B., Trentacosta, C. J., & McLear, C. (2014). Client preferences affect treatment satisfaction, completion, and clinical outcome: A meta-analysis. *Clinical psychology review*, 34(6), 506–517.
Magistretti, P., & Ansermet, F. (2010). *Neurosciences et psychanalyse*. Paris: Odile Jacob.
Makari, G. (2008). *Revolution in mind: The creation of psychoanalysis*. London: Duckworth Press.

Moser, U., & von Zeppelin, I. (1996). Der geträumte Traum. *Wie Träume entstehen und sich verändern.* Stuttgart: Kohlhammer.

Rolland, J-C. (2020). *Langue et psyché. Instantanés métapsychologiques.* Paris: Éditions d'Ithaque.

Shedler, J. (2010). The efficacy of psychodynamic psychotherapy. *American Psychologist*, 65(2), 98–109.

Shedler, J. (2018). Where is the evidence for "evidence-based" therapy?. *Psychiatric Clinics*, 41(2), 319–329.

Siclari, F., Valli, K. & Arnulf, I. (2020). Dreams and nightmares in healthy adults and in patients with sleep and neurological disorders. *Lancet Neurology*, 19(10), 849–859.

Steinert, C., Hofmann, M., Kruse, J., & Leichsenring, F. (2014). Relapse rates after psychotherapy for depression – stable long-term effects? A meta-analysis. *Journal of Affective Disorders*, 168, 107–118.

Steinmair, D., & Löffler-Stastka, H. (2021). The emerging role of interdisciplinarity in clinical psychoanalysis. *Frontiers in Psychology*, 12, 1603.

Windle, E., Tee, H., Sabitova, A., Jovanovic, N., Priebe, S., & Carr, C. (2020). Association of patient treatment preference with dropout and clinical outcomes in adult psychosocial mental health interventions: A systematic review and meta-analysis. *JAMA Psychiatry*, 77(3), 294–302.

14 Memory re-consolidation and dreaming

Shadows of the night

Tamara Fischmann, Marianne Leuzinger-Bohleber and Gilles Ambresin

Introduction: changes in dreams – an indicator for transformations in the inner world of patients during psychoanalyses

Whether and how psychoanalysis contributes to change in chronically depressed patients remains a central question not only for the affected individuals and their families, but also for the legitimacy of psychoanalytic treatments in today's health-care system. As discussed in the introduction to this volume, the attempt to also capture such change empirically raises complex epistemological and methodological challenges, which have been one reason why to this day many practicing psychoanalysts remain skeptical of comparative outcome studies in psychotherapy. For example, they object to the fact that in many comparative psychotherapy studies, including the LAC Depression Study, the main criterion of therapeutic success is defined as self- and blind-assessments of the reduction of depressive symptoms, e.g. by using questionnaires like the Beck's Depression Inventory (cf. e.g. Leuzinger-Bohleber et al., 2019). As we discussed in the previous chapter, this was one reason why we have chosen a multi-perspective approach to look at the therapeutic outcome in the follow-up study to the LAC study, the MODE study. Psychological outcome criteria are compared with neurobiological and psychoanalytic indicators of change in a complementary and contrasting manner.

With this design and research aims we draw on a long tradition of psychoanalytic outcome research. Already in the 1980s, Leuzinger-Bohleber was able to show, on the basis of five aggregated single case studies that the manifest dreams of the first compared to the last hundred therapy sessions in long psychoanalyses, differed systematically (Leuzinger-Bohleber, 1989; 2012). The manifest dreams – according to the evaluations of patients, their analysts, and independent observers – "successful" psychoanalyses show a wider range of affects, more successful problem solving with a more active dream self, fewer nightmares and fewer dreams in which the dream self is in a passive position. These findings were replicated by Kächele and his research group (Kächele et al., 2006). Our research group has also conducted a number of initial studies in which these changes in dreams have also been investigated by neurobiological instruments (see e.g., Fischmann, Leuzinger-Bohleber, &

DOI: 10.4324/9781003279297-14

Kächele, 2012; Fischmann, Russ, & Leuzinger-Bohleber, 2013). We have widely discussed the interesting but challenging epistemological and methodological topics connected to such interdisciplinary research endeavors (see e.g., Fischmann et al., 2012; Fischmann & Leuzinger-Bohleber, 2017; Fischmann et al., 2015; Leuzinger-Bohleber et al., 2015; Leuzinger-Bohleber & Fischmann, 2017).

In the following section we would like to elaborate newer conceptual ideas which seem fascinating and enlightening as theoretical backgrounds for the empirical investigation of the transformation of manifest dreams. The first section comprises some studies on memory consolidation. In the section thereafter we discuss an integrative dream generating model by Moser and von Zeppelin (1996). Based on this model these authors and their research group have developed a new empirical rating system for evaluating changes of manifest dreams during psychoanalyses (see e.g., Moser & Hortig, 2019).

Freud's dream theory and memory consolidation

Memory formation is often understood as having three stages: encoding – storage – retrieval, all of which are accompanied by biological changes. One interesting question connected to this process, apart from the differentiation of the different types of memories, is that the physical changes underlying the encoding and processing of information after a discrete event remain in a fragile or rather labile state for some time before the memory is consolidated.

Memory consolidation is a diverse process: for one there is the initial gene expression-dependent phase which lasts from several hours up to 1–2 days, after which a memory becomes consolidated and stable. Thereafter there is also a retrieval-dependent fragility of memory mediated by trace rearrangement among brain regions in which, when reactivated, memory becomes fragile once more and can be altered again and then re-stabilized over a much longer period of time. The latter process has been defined as memory re-consolidation (Alberini, Johnson, & Ye, 2013; Nader & Einarsson, 2010; Sara, 2010; Squire, 2009; Squire et al., 2015).

Since memory becomes labile after retrieval, this challenges the question why does this happen? One hypothesis is that through this process the memory may be updated since new information is integrated into the background of the past (Sara, 2000a; Dudai & Eisenberg, 2004). Another hypothesis proposes that re-consolidation is necessary so that memory can become stronger and longer lasting (Sara, 2000b). Based on current knowledge, the function of re-consolidation is to mediate memory strengthening and prevent forgetting of the same memory trace.

Thus, time passage is essential for memory formation and storage and worthwhile to note is that implicit or explicit events will most likely reactivate memory traces, where implicit activations will usually occur during rest and sleep.

As for memory and dreaming it is important to note that in dreaming the same dopaminergic (SEEKING) system is active as in purposive waking life (see e.g., Panksepp, 2004; Solms, 2021). But, in sleep the sensory input is attended to minimally in order to guard and ensure sleep. This frees the brain to minimize complexity in REM dreaming and by this assumedly resolves otherwise disruptive (emotional) conflicts.

Let us consider another interesting hypothesis, namely what Hobson et al. (Hobson, Hong, & Friston, 2014) pointed out in an interesting paper on consciousness and dreaming – that dreaming seems to have a predictive aspect. As many dream researchers have found, dreaming is a simulator of the world. What we call waking life is a form of online dreaming (Metzinger, 2013, p. 140). Hobson et al. stated that dreaming tells waking what to expect. Waking verifies or refuses those expectations (Hobson et al., 2014, p. 2). This could mean that remembering is part of dreaming. While waking memory as well as orientation are weakened in dreaming and logical inference is virtually impossible in dreaming, dreaming is associated with a narrower range but a greater depth of emotions than waking. Taking all these differences between waking and dreaming, it seems as if "dreaming were a warm-up exercise for the game of waking" (Hobson et al., 2014, p. 2).

Let us return for a moment to Freud and his dream theory (Freud, 1900). In his model of dream formation, Freud assumed that impingements from inside (major needs) or outside (life situation, day residue) cause us to dream. This aspect nicely relates to Friston's concept of free energy (FE; Friston, 2012). Friston hypothesizes that the brain operates to minimize FE caused by sensory impingements of unpredicted stimuli. And like Freud who assumed major needs or biological imperatives to reflect such impingements, Friston proposes that these sensory impingements reflect compliance with biological imperatives, creating a "demand for work" (Freud, 1915) to produce "specific actions" or to put it in Friston's words "an imperative to minimize prediction error … through action" (Friston, 2012, p. 248). For both Freud and Friston, when such sensory impingements are felt, they put a demand on our brain to embody a representation of these sensory impingements including representations of the "bodily ego" (Freud, 1923) or as Friston would term it the "agent's body". These bodily representations are initially met by an innate generation of a prior virtual version of reality, i.e., a phantasy of reality, which will subsequently be modified by experience.

Now there is another interesting phenomenon, namely that REM especially has a neurodevelopmental function. In utero at 30 weeks of gestational age an infant is already spending most of its time in REM (Hobson & Friston, 2012; see Figure 14.1) and one might conclude that humans are *genetically endowed with an innate virtual reality generator, whose working is most clearly revealed in [REM] dreaming.*

We might say from here, that Freud's primary process – preponderant in dreams – and the virtual reality generator are innate producers of imaginary prior belief and/or experience. According to Freud this primary process is "in the apparatus first", which could be termed in Friston's words as prior beliefs. Freud describes perception, learning, and action as secondary processes prepared by the innate primary process, set into motion by the sensory impact of birth.

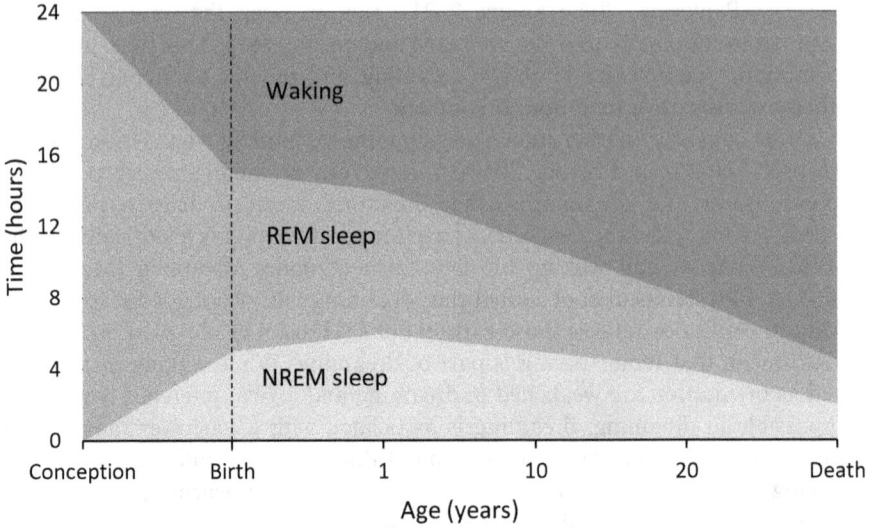

Figure 14.1 Human sleep and age. The predominance of rapid eye movement (REM) sleep in the last trimester of pregnancy (after conception) and in the first year of life progressively declines as waking time increases. Despite its early decrease, REM sleep continues to occur for about 1.5 hours per day throughout life.

Dream consciousness thus precedes waking consciousness by months in utero and in adult life by hours.

This is underscored by the notion of a virtual reality model creator in dreaming which is counterbalanced by a generative model in waking life. Dreaming and REM, considered in this way, play a major role in conscious inference, in conscious experience and understanding of what real life teaches us thru experience. Dreams phenomenologically perform a perceptual synthesis by testing real life experiences virtually (in dreams) creating a generalizable generative model of the world, which is thereafter tested in conscious waking life for its functionability.

Perceptually informed belief and action thus replace virtual reality (phantasy) in waking life.

As memory and the wake–sleep cycle become established after birth, the unconstrained production of phantasy/virtual reality are relegated to dreaming, where it continues to play a role in minimizing free energy (FE). Minimizing FE is essential because it prevents us from making mistakes. The less FE is available, the less prediction errors we make regarding our coping. The more complex our model of life becomes, i.e., the way we understand what happens in our lives, which is what we are trying to do in therapy, the more FE is bound. This complexity on the other hand may be considered to be a weakness, as the more complex our models become, the more difficult they are to master in our everyday lives. Dreaming offers a solution here as it helps us to minimize FE while simultaneously reducing complexity, simply by creating a fantasized world of how things could work. Complexity is reduced in dreams, because in dreams everything is possible and must not be complex. Now let's see how this is so.

If we assume that what arouses dreaming especially in REM is a non-sensory source, since there is sensorimotor attenuation during REM; we may assume further that such a non-sensory source of FE-arousing data must be emotions, which inevitably attend REM and which in turn may be assumed to be part of consolidation/re-consolidation of memory. This again accords with Freud's dreamwork operating to condense emotionally significant elements from a range of memories associated with the dream. Translated to neuroscience language: what Freud describes as condensation appears to reflect a collection of data over remembered and associated arousals of amygdala-related emotion that could be compared to the saccadic collection of sensory data in waking. So, if we really dare to assume that associated remembered arousals are data of fictive perceptual experiences, then dreaming serves to unify, predict, and inhibit arousals, thereby minimizing FE (as emotional conflict/complexity) in a way closely analogous to the realistic perceptual experiences of waking, which in turn serves memory consolidation (Rasch & Born, 2013; Palombo, 1978).

To summarize the role of dreaming in memory re-consolidation: sleep consists of cyclically alternating NREM- and REM-sleep cycles. Slow oscillations in the NREM-SWS (Slow Wave Sleep) effect the downscaling of synaptic homeostasis, while hippocampal sharp wave ripples activate large areas of the cortex, transferring recent memories from the hippocampus to the cortical areas appropriate for long-term storage. Within this sleep-cycle, as SWS yields to REM, memories are reactivated and the reactivated memories then become labile so that together with the re-aroused emotions they can be re-consolidated under the impact of dreaming in a new and emotionally revised integration of emotion and declarative content (Van der Helm et al., 2011; Genzel et al., 2015). Dreams thus evidently play a complexity-reducing role during consolidation/re-consolidation of memory. REM dreaming performs an "emotional valence re-evaluation and adjustment" in updating and revising the amygdala-related emotions associated with memory (Van der Helm et al., 2011; Genzel et al., 2015; see also (Gujar et al., 2011; Goldstein & Walker, 2014).

We can therefore expect that complexity reduction occurs together with the updating of the emotional meaning of old memories. Dreaming and especially REM with its emotional significance and plasticity-inducing circumstances has a powerful revisionary effect on cortically embodied long-term memories during sleep where those memories are hence updated, and their declarative content strengthened. In other words, REM dreaming maintains the accuracy together with the reduction of emotional complexity of memories and plays a role in consolidation of memories.

Recent work on REM dreaming (Van der Helm et al., 2011; Genzel at al., 2015) revealed dreaming to perform emotional valence re-evaluation and adjustment in updating and revising the amygdala-related emotions associated with memory. From what we have reported so far, it would be safe to assume that complexity reduction would occur together with the updating of the emotional significance of old memories and that the vivid experiences of dreaming during plasticity-inducing REM could have a powerful revisionary effect on the emotional significance of cortically embodied long-term memories undergoing updating in sleep while strengthening their declarative content. As Osan et al. (Osan, Tort, & Amaral, 2011) have pointed out, only similar contextual re-exposure or radical different contextual re-exposure induce re-consolidation, making dreaming with its real-life vividness and radical different bizarreness an appropriate candidate for re-consolidation (Zhao, Li, & Li, 2018).

Having said all this, we would like to turn to the manifest dream, i.e., the dream remembered as a candidate for memory consolidation and re-consolidation. What do we know? As said before, when SWS yields to REM, memories are reactivated and those memories become labile so that they together with the reactivated emotions can be re-consolidated; thus we may conclude that REM dreaming performs emotional re-evaluation of memories. We may assume, that the manifest dream (the dream remembered) is caused by the arousal of the same memories and emotions of day-residues that were active on the day of the dream and we may regard the manifest dream as working to alter some of these emotions during their arousal.

Manifest dreams, memory re-consolidation and the dream-generation-model (Moser & von Zeppelin, 1996)

If we consider the manifest dream to be a candidate for re-consolidation, we would of course like to investigate whether and how we will find indicators for memory consolidation processes in the manifest dream. And here another dream theory comes into play. In their "dream-generation-model" Moser and von Zeppelin (Moser & von Zeppelin, 1996) proposed that current concerns (day residues) activate so-called dream complexes in which the entire information of unresolved conflicts (= Focal Conflict (FC)) and traumatic situations are contained and there represented (see Figure 14.2).

The dream looks for solutions or the best possible adaptations to such dream complexes. A dream, which is normally pictorial, consists of at least one situation produced by a dream-organizer. According to Moser, dream-organization can be regarded as a number of affective–cognitive procedures that generate a micro-world – the dream – and control its course. Within this system, the dream complex serves as a kind of template for the dream-organization. Viewed in this way, the dream complex consists of one or more complexes stored in long-term memory that have arisen from conflictual and/or traumatic experiences, which manifest themselves in introjects. It is characteristic for these introjects that on the one hand they are closely linked to the triggering environmental stimuli and on the other hand they are structurally similar to the stored situations of the complex (memory).

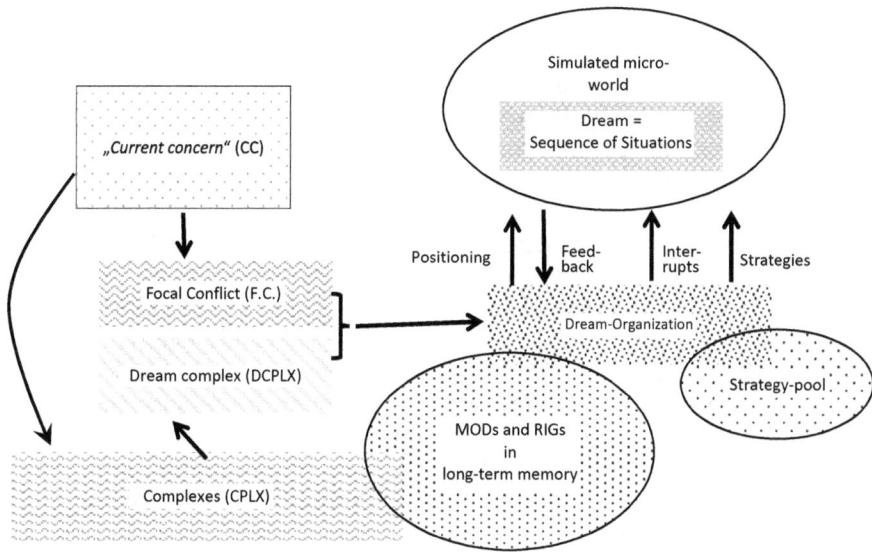

Figure 14.2 Dream-generation model.

Conflictual complexes are isolated areas of bundled desires, RIGs (General-ized Interaction Reactions) and MODs (Object-relation Models), whereby areas of unbound affective information arise, because they exist separately from the remaining memory content (are repressed or have never been formulated at all and are thus dissociated). Affects within such areas are connected to each other (by so-called k-lines). To resolve these conflictual complexes (i.e., make them accessible to memory – again), it is necessary to connect the affective information with the relationship reality so that they can become perceivable, declarative, alive, and accessible.

This is exactly what dreams try to do, because their function is to find solutions for isolated, dissociated complexes. The sought-after solution of this task, namely, to reintegrate the isolated complexes into our psychic reality, to make them declarative is determined by an innate need for security and a desire to be involved. Moser and von Zeppelin refer to these principles, which regulate the organization of dreams, as the principle of security and involve-ment. The control within the dream event by these two principles can be imagined as a kind of temperature regulation. If it gets too hot – i.e., if the affective temperature rises – the dreamer will strive for more security – to cool down – and will be less inclined to get involved.

As can be seen from this dream theory, memory and affects play a central role in solving conflictual complexes, which can only be solved if they can be *Re-Transcribed* into a relationship reality. This re-transcription is very similar to what has been claimed for emotional re-evaluation processes of memories during dreaming.

Moser and Hortig (2019) have developed a sophisticated method – the ZDPCS (Zurich Dream Process Coding System) – to identify indicators for these affective change processes in the manifest dream – it being the dream remembered.

Changes of affect regulation within dreams are crucial indicators that the dreamer's ability to approach conflictual themes is increasing. As unconscious, non-declarative memory content cannot be retrieved and thought about – as it is non-declarative – the only way for disturbing memories to come to consciousness is via affects connected to these memories. This may be interpreted as a beginning of consolidation of something formerly unthinkable. Within the ZDPCS this may be observed for one via fewer interruptions and cognitive processes (CPs) between situations within a dream. Each interruption of a dream-scene indicates that the dream is getting emotionally too "hot", i.e., the dream approaches areas of unresolved conflictual complexes interconnected by unbound, painful affects. With each dream-scene the dreamer searches to resolve this complex by either introducing new helpful objects (involvement principle) or by distancing himself (security principle). In general, one could say that the fewer interruptions a dream contains, and the more interactions that are possible within a dream, the closer the dreamer comes to solving his or her conflictual complexes. In this way, dreams reveal that new memory traces that are less conflictual and less emotionally painful are consolidated. This is only possible in dreams, as dreams are governed by primary process thinking and the pleasure principle. In mental activity of the primary process there is free, uninhibited flow of psychic energy from one idea to another, without regard for logic or reality dominated by the pleasure principle. It provides hallucinatory fulfillment of wishes, which is what dreaming does.

To summarize: memories can be changed when they are labile and in a fragile state. That is the case when they are reactivated implicitly or explicitly. They can then be re-consolidated. Conflictual and traumatic memories are usually associated with intense painful emotions. It is those emotions that are there all the time, the actual event that caused them is often dissociated and cannot be declared – it is unconscious. These dissociated traumatic memories are very disturbing because we cannot make sense of them, we cannot integrate them into our psychic reality, but we feel them all the time. What we try to do in psychoanalysis is to reach out to these memories and make sense of them, make them bearable and thinkable, by creating more tolerable new memory traces.

The psychic change that goes hand in hand with this can be seen clinically but also empirically. One indicator for this psychic change is dreams, which we have tried to explain by drawing on Freud's dream theory, which we have related to Friston's FE principle, to explain how this might happen: in REM-dreaming we create virtual realities in the search for solutions of unbound emotions, trying to bind them back into our psychic reality. In waking life, we test those virtual reality models, making generative reality models that help us to get through life. The economic advantage of this is that in dreams we bind FE and reduce complexity more easily and finding a solution is more readily possible.

We have then turned to another dream theory, that of Moser and von Zeppelin, where we can find indicators of such changes in the manifest dreams.

The exciting part is that with all this knowledge gathered on memory consolidation and re-consolidation in dreaming, we can feel more confident to use dreams as indicators of change during times of crisis, in psychotherapies and experimental studies of psychic change.

Dreams are not only subjective narratives, they are indeed memories sometimes re-consolidated, sometimes newly consolidated, and always emotionally reevaluated – i.e., virtual reality models to be tested in waking life to create a generative reality model of the world with which we may be able to cope better in life.

Concluding remarks

Dreams are still considered the "Via Regia to the unconscious" today. Referring to recent contributions to the concept of memory re-consolidation we have discussed that dreams offer a unique possibility to re-evaluate and adjust memories of emotionally significant and often traumatic conflict situations by updating and revising the emotions related to these memories and reducing their complexity to consolidate new memory traces or re-consolidate old ones thus creating virtual reality models to then be tested in real life situations to cope better. This view is one reason why changes in manifest dreams can be seen as psychoanalytically interesting indicators for transformations that have taken place in psychoanalyses and have therefore also been empirically studied as genuine psychoanalytic criteria for changes that have taken place in psychoanalyses (cf. Leuzinger-Bohleber, 1989, 2012; Fischmann et al., 2013). The MODE study builds on these traditions (cf. Ambresin et al., Chapter 13 in this volume). It uses the elaborated ZDPCS (Zurich Dream Process Coding System) presented in this paper to systematically investigate such changes in chronically depressed, early traumatized patients during low- and high-frequency psychoanalyses (see Fischmann & Leuzinger-Bohleber, 2018; Fischmann, Ambresin, & Leuzinger-Bohleber, 2021).

References

Alberini, C. M., Johnson, S. A., & Ye, X. (2013). Memory reconsolidation: Lingering consolidation and the dynamic memory trace. In: C. M. Alberini (Ed.), *Memory reconsolidation* (pp. 81–117). Amsterdam: Elsevier.

Dudai, Y., & Eisenberg, M. (2004). Rites of passage of the engram: Reconsolidation and the lingering consolidation hypothesis. *Neuron*, 44(1), 93–100.

Fischmann, T., Ambresin, G., & Leuzinger-Bohleber, M. (2021). Dreams and trauma changes in the manifest dreams in psychoanalytic treatments: A psychoanalytic outcome measure. *Frontiers in Psychology*, 12, 1–8.

Fischmann, T., & Leuzinger-Bohleber, M. (2017). Veränderungen von Träumen als Indikatoren für Therapieerfolg. *Trauma—Zeitschrift Für Psychotraumatologie Und Ihre Anwendungen*, 15(2), 80–89.

Fischmann, T., & Leuzinger-Bohleber, M. (2018). Dreams. In: H. Böker, P. Hartwich, & G. Northoff (Eds.), *Neuropsychodynamic Psychiatry* (pp. 137–155). New York: Springer.

Fischmann, T., Leuzinger-Bohleber, M., & Kächele, H. (2012). Traumforschung in der Psychoanalyse: Klinische Studien, Traumserien, extraklinische Forschung im Labor. *Psyche*, 66(9–10), 833–861.

Fischmann, T., Leuzinger-Bohleber, M., Schött, M., & Russ, M. (2015). Traum und psychische Transformationsprozesse in Psychoanalysen: ein Dialog zwischen Psychoanalyse und Neurowissenschaften In: M. Leuzinger-Bohleber, T. Fischmann, H. Böker, G. Northoff, & M. Solms (Eds.), *Psychoanalyse und Neurowissenschaften* (pp. 185–218). Stuttgart: Kohlhammer.

Fischmann, T., Russ, M., Baehr, T., Stirn, A., & Leuzinger-Bohleber, M. (2012). Changes in dreams of chronic depressed patients the Frankfurt fMRI/EEG study (FRED). In: P. Fonagy, H. Kächele, M. Leuzinger-Bohleber, & D. Taylor (Eds.), *The significance of dreams: Bridging clinical and extraclinical research in psychoanalysis* (pp. 157–181). London: Karnac Books.

Fischmann, T., Russ, M. O., & Leuzinger-Bohleber, M. (2013). Trauma, dream, and psychic change in psychoanalyses: a dialog between psychoanalysis and the neurosciences. *Frontiers in Human Neuroscience*, 7, article 877. doi:10.3389/fnhum.2013.00877.

Freud, S. (1900). Die Methode der Traumdeutung. In: *Gesammelte Werke: II/III: Die Traumdeutung über den Traum* (pp. 100–126). Frankfurt am Main: Fischer Taschenbuch Verlag, 1999.

Freud, S. (1915). Instincts and their vicissitudes. In: *The standard edition of the complete psychological works of Sigmund Freud*, Volume XIV (1914–1916): On the history of the psycho-analytic movement, papers on metapsychology and other works (pp. 109–140).

Freud, S. (1923). *The ego and the id*. London: Hogarth Press and Institute of Psycho-Analysis.

Friston, K. (2012). Prediction, perception and agency. *International Journal of Psychophysiology*, 83(2), 248–252.

Genzel, L., Spoormaker, V., Konrad, B., & Dresler, M. (2015). The role of rapid eye movement sleep for amygdala-related memory processing. *Neurobiology of Learning and Memory*, 122, 110–121.

Goldstein, A. N., & Walker, M. P. (2014). The role of sleep in emotional brain function. *Annual Review of Clinical Psychology*, 10, 679–708.

Gujar, N., McDonald, S. A., Nishida, M., & Walker, M. P. (2011). A role for REM sleep in recalibrating the sensitivity of the human brain to specific emotions. *Cerebral Cortex*, 21(1), 115–123.

Hobson, J. A., & Friston, K. J. (2012). Waking and dreaming consciousness: Neurobiological and functional considerations. *Progress in Neurobiology*, 98(1), 82–98.

Hobson, J. A., Hong, C. C.-H., & Friston, K. J. (2014). Virtual reality and consciousness inference in dreaming. *Frontiers in Psychology*, 5, 1133.

Kächele, H., Leuzinger-Bohleber, M., Buchheim, A., & Thomä, H. (2006). Amalie X: ein deutscher Musterfall (Ebene I und Ebene II). In: H. Thomä & H. Kächele (Eds.), *Psychoanalytische Therapie: Forschung* (pp. 121–174). Heidelberg: Springer.

Leuzinger-Bohleber, M. (1989). *Veränderung kognitiver problemlösender Prozesse in Psychoanalysen* (Vol. 2: *Fünf aggregierte Einzelfälle*). Ulm: PSZ Verlag (Springer).

Leuzinger-Bohleber, M. (2012). Changes in dreams: From a psychoanalysis with a traumatised, chronic depressed patient. In: P. Fonagy, H. Kächele, M. Leuzinger-

Bohleber, & D. Taylor (Eds.), *The significance of dreams: Bridging clinical and extraclinical research in psychoanalysis* (pp. 49–85). London: Karnac Books.

Leuzinger-Bohleber, M., Böker, H., Fischmann, T., Northoff, G., & Solms, M. (2015). *Psychoanalyse und Neurowissenschaften: Chancen-Grenzen-Kontroversen*. Stuttgart: Kohlhammer Verlag.

Leuzinger-Bohleber, M., & Fischmann, T. (2017). Veränderungen von Träumen als Indikatoren für Therapieerfolg. Teil 1: Manifeste Trauminhalte von traumatisierten Patienten in Psychoanalysen. Trauma. *Zeitschrift für Psychotraumatologie und ihre Anwendungen*, 15(2), 70–80.

Leuzinger-Bohleber, M., Kaufhold, J., Kallenbach, L., Negele, A., Ernst, M., Keller, W., ... Beutel, M. (2019). How to measure sustained psychic transformations in long-term treatments of chronically depressed patients: Symptomatic and structural changes in the LAC Depression Study of the outcome of cognitive-behavioural and psychoanalytic long-term treatments. *The International Journal of Psychoanalysis*, 100(1), 99–127.

Metzinger, T. K. (2013). Why are dreams interesting for philosophers? The example of minimal phenomenal selfhood, plus an agenda for future research1. *Frontiers in Psychology*, 4, 746.

Moser, U., & Hortig, V. (2019). Mikrowelt Traum. *Affektregulierung und Reflexion*. Frankfurt a. M.: Brandes & Apsel.

Moser, U., & von Zeppelin, I. (1996). *Der geträumte Traum: wie Träume entstehen und sich verändern*. Stuttgart: Kohlhammer.

Nader, K., & Einarsson, E. Ö. (2010). Memory reconsolidation: an update. *Annals of the New York Academy of Sciences*, 1191(1), 27–41.

Osan, R., Tort, A. B., & Amaral, O. B. (2011). A mismatch-based model for memory reconsolidation and extinction in attractor networks. *PloS One*, 6(8), e23113.

Palombo, S. R. (1978). The adaptive function of dreams. *Psychoanalysis and Contemporary Thought*, 1(4), 443–476.

Panksepp, J. (2004). *Affective neuroscience: The foundations of human and animal emotions*: New York, NY: Oxford University Press.

Rasch, B., & Born, J. (2013). About sleep's role in memory. *Physiological Reviews*, 93, 681–766.

Sara, S. J. (2000a). Retrieval and reconsolidation: Toward a neurobiology of remembering. *Learning & Memory*, 7(2), 73–84.

Sara, S. J. (2000b). Strengthening the shaky trace through retrieval. *Nature Reviews Neuroscience*, 1(3), 212–213.

Sara, S. J. (2010). Reactivation, retrieval, replay and reconsolidation in and out of sleep: Connecting the dots. *Frontiers in Behavioral Neuroscience*, 4, 185.

Solms, M. (2021). *The hidden spring: A journey to the source of consciousness*. New York, NY: WW Norton.

Squire, L. R. (2009). Memory and brain systems: 1969–2009. *Journal of Neuroscience*, 29(41), 12711–12716.

Squire, L. R., Genzel, L., Wixted, J. T., & Morris, R. G. (2015). Memory consolidation. *Cold Spring Harbor Perspectives in Biology*, 7(8), a021766.

Van der Helm, E., Yao, J., Dutt, S., Rao, V., Saletin, J. M., & Walker, M. P. (2011). REM sleep depotentiates amygdala activity to previous emotional experiences. *Current Biology*, 21(23), 2029–2032.

Zhao, H., Li, D., & Li, X. (2018). Relationship between dreaming and memory reconsolidation. *Brain Science Advances*, 4(2), 118–130.

15 Depression in neuropsychoanalysis
Why does depression feel bad?

Mark Solms

Sometimes it is necessary to review the basics in order to see the big picture, and there are some very basic things that I would like to review in this chapter. Reading the subtitle of my chapter, which is based on earlier papers (Watt & Panksepp, 2009; Solms & Panksepp, 2010; Zellner et al., 2011), readers might think I am asking a silly question. However, this is a question that we really do need to ask, because in psychiatry today it is a question that is not even considered. *Why* the patient feels what they are feeling, what the feeling *means* (psychologically), and what the feeling *does* (causally), are not serious questions in contemporary psychiatry.

In psychoanalysis, we believe that feelings exist for a reason (Solms, 2018). They are not epiphenomena; they are not something that is just 'nice to have', added onto the brain's *real* workings. Feelings are absolutely central to how the brain works. If we don't take account of feelings, we will never understand the brain. Sentience is *the* distinguishing property of the brain; it is what sets it apart from all other organs. This is what Freud thought. But in academic psychology and psychiatry through the 20th century, other ideas took hold. Now, in the 21st century, we in neuropsychoanalysis want to return to Freud's original idea, taking account of what has been learnt by other mental-science disciplines in the intervening century. That is why we must consider such simple questions afresh.

Let us take an extremely basic example. If you meet a friend and she looks sad, that means something. It tells you something about what is going on inside her, and it gives you an indication as to how she might respond to you (i.e., it has causal implications.) She will behave differently if she is sad, from how she might behave if she were angry or anxious. This is because different feelings *mean* different things, and they make people *do* different things. Nothing could be more obvious. Right?

Well, let us see what the experts think …

Behaviourism

This was the approach to the mind that replaced psychoanalysis in the academic psychology of the mid-20th century. Freud (1940) wrote that conscious

DOI: 10.4324/9781003279297-15

feeling was "the most unique characteristic" of the part of nature that we call the mind – "a fact without parallel". He then added:

> one extreme line of thought, exemplified in the American doctrine of beha-viourism, thinks it possible to construct a psychology which disregards this fundamental fact!

(Freud, 1940, p. 157)

It is well known why behaviourists wanted to construct a science of the mind that disregarded its most unique characteristic. Consciousness cannot be observed externally; it is not amenable to *objective* scrutiny. Consciousness is for that reason an embarrassment to science, the ideal of which is objective fact over subjective experience. The behaviourists, who wanted to treat the mind as if it were no different from any other part of nature, therefore ruled subjectivity out of court, and limited scientific psychology to the study of the externally observable *outputs* of the mind – to the study of *behaviour*. Objec-tive experimental manipulations ('stimuli') could then be used to discover the causal mechanisms of behavioural 'responses'. In this way, the intervening variables (conceptualized as *learning*) became the only valid objects of psychological science.

Not surprisingly, a school of thought predicated on the assumption that the mind consists in nothing but learning (e.g., depression is a learnt response), and disregards all the mental phenomena that we "know immediately and from our most personal experience" (Freud, ibid.), was doomed to failure. To deny the causal influence on behaviour of conscious states (like feelings) is to deny the obvious. If one says: that person committed suicide because he could not stand the pain any longer, one is describing the simple causal power of the unfortunate person's feelings. If one were to try to reframe such causal rela-tions so as to exclude the feelings, and base them on learning alone, one would be doing obvious violence to the actual scientific facts.

Cognitive science

Thankfully, therefore, in the last quarter of the 20th century, realism tri-umphed over fundamentalism, and feelings found their way back into psy-chological science. Even though consciousness still cannot be observed directly, or objectively, cognitive scientists today are nevertheless willing to acknowledge its *existence* in their experimental subjects, and on this basis to infer the causal mechanisms by which conscious states influence behaviours – in much the same way as the behaviourists were willing to infer the causal mechanisms of learning.

Or are they?

The mechanisms of consciousness may be ontologically equivalent to those of learning (or anything else in the mind) but the *mechanisms* of conscious-ness differ in fundamental respects from consciousness *itself*. Mechanisms of all kinds are abstractions, *inferred* from experience;[1] they are not experiences themselves. The mechanisms of consciousness, like all other mechanisms, therefore present no special problems for science; they, too, can be described from an objective standpoint, from the third-person point of view, as *functions*. But this excludes the 'fundamental fact' of felt consciousness, namely that we experience it directly.

Is consciousness not perhaps still an embarrassment to science; do cognitive scientists today not perhaps still think it possible to construct a psychology which disregards the *causal* role of feelings – this uniquely subjective characteristic of the mind – the fundamental characteristic of this part of nature?

Cognitive neuroscience

It is, in my view, no accident that the apparent re-admittance of consciousness to psychology coincided with advances in the neurosciences which made it possible to study the physiological correlates of almost any mental state. By shifting the focus of their research efforts to the *physical correlates* of consciousness, neuroscientists were able to pay lip service to its existence without having to trouble themselves too much with its intrinsically subjective nature – with the original source of the embarrassment.

Small wonder, then, that so many behaviourists made such a seamless transition to the new paradigm. As Freud (ibid.) put it:

> There would thus be no alternative left to assuming that there are physical or somatic processes which are concomitant with the psychical ones and which we should necessarily have to recognize as more complete than the psychical sequences [... Then] it of course becomes plausible to lay the stress in psychology on those somatic processes, to see in them the true essence of what is psychical.

To seek the essence of what is psychical in something which lacks its most unique property is surely to look in the wrong place. But this does not mean that we must abandon reality. Nor does it mean (today) that the brain is the wrong place to seek an understanding of consciousness. It means only that we must admit that consciousness actually exists, that it is a property of nature, that it is a property of the part of nature called the brain, and that this property is no less real and no less causally efficacious than any other natural properties. This in turn means that we must recognize that the brain is not quite the same as every other part of nature. The brain has some special properties, and central among these is feeling. As a consequence of it being conscious, the brain behaves differently from most other things, even from other bodily organs.

As far as I can tell, despite appearances, these views are still not generally accepted, or at least they are not generally incorporated into the current theoretical paradigms of cognitive neuroscience. In fact, the very power of cognitive neuroscience seems to be that it treats the organ of the mind as if it were no different from any other bodily organ, indeed from any other complex mechanism – living or dead.

As Oliver Sacks put it:

> Neuropsychology, like classical neurology, aims to be entirely objective, and its great power, its advances, come from just this. But a living creature, and especially a human being, is firstand last active – a subject, not an object. It is precisely the subject, the living 'I', which is being excluded. Neuropsychology is admirable, but it excludes the psyche – it excludes the experiencing, active, living 'I'.
>
> (Sacks, 1984, p. 164)

Biological psychiatry

The baneful consequences of this continued neglect of the fundamental fact of consciousness have been even more evident in the field of biological psychiatry than in cognitive neuroscience. This is perhaps not surprising, because psychiatry is all about feelings. How else does it differ from neurology?

In biological psychiatry today, if one says: the patient committed suicide because he could not stand the pain any longer, one seems to mean: the patient thought he was committing suicide because he could not stand the pain any longer, but *really* he was committing suicide because his serotonin levels were depleted (or something like that). The point is: what the patient says, thinks or feels may be left out of the scientific account; feelings evidently are not part of the actual causal chain of events. They are just a layperson's translation of the real state of affairs in the brain. This is just fundamentalism.

Depression in biological psychiatry

I shall now illustrate this problem in modern psychiatry with reference to our particular question, namely: why depression feels bad.

As I have said, this question is not even posed in biological psychiatry. It is not posed because what depression feels like does not matter in contemporary psychiatric science. This is evidently because feelings in general do not matter. What matters in biological psychiatry, no less than cognitive neuroscience, is the physical correlates of the feelings. This approach is based on a serious misconception of how the brain works, which will almost inevitably lead to grave mistakes. In their haste to avoid the embarrassingly subjective phenomena of depression, psychiatric researchers have in recent decades focused on all sorts of things that correlate with depression, or facilitate it, or contextualize it – and the neural mechanisms of those things – rather than depression itself.

The main focus of depression research for the past few decades has been the neurophysiological mechanisms of serotonin depletion (Schildkraut, 1965; Harro & Oreland, 2001), including the neurotrophic effects of this depletion

(Koziek et al., 2008), the neuroendocrinological mechanisms of stress (which has similar neurotrophic consequences) (De Kloet et al., 2005), the neuroimmunological equivalents of these mechanisms (McEwen, 2007), their interactions with sleep mechanisms (Zupancic & Guilleminault, 2006), their genetic underpinnings (Levinson, 2006), and so on. These research programmes have evidently been followed because the mechanisms of serotonin depletion (and its cognates) are eminently tractable scientific problems – notwithstanding the fact that they have nothing to do with actually researching depressive feelings.

The reason these programs have been followed cannot possibly be because the researchers concerned seriously thought that depressive feelings (let alone major depression) are actually caused by low levels of serotonin. There is not a shred of evidence for that. In fact, it is well established that experimental depletion of brain serotonin does not cause depression (Delgado et al., 1990). Nor was there ever any reason to believe that serotonin would play any such specific causal role in depressive mood. Serotonin is a general-purpose modulator of moods and emotions, not only of depressive ones (Berger, Gray & Roth, 2009). It is probably for this reason that SSRIs are used to treat not only depression but also a host of other emotional troubles, such as panic attacks and obsessive compulsive disorder. This is also probably the reason why SSRIs do not work in so many cases of depression, and why they work only partially or temporarily in the vast majority of cases (cf. STAR*D findings). The same applies to the various cascades associated with serotonin depletion: stress or inflammation or hippocampal shrinkage. None of these things has a specific causal relationship with depression. They are too general; 'too much' of an explanation. Their main attraction is only that they are scientifically tractable and therefore scientifically respectable, objective mechanisms.

In summary, it is clear that although the mechanisms of serotonin depletion and its cognates correlate with or facilitate or contextualize depression, something else – something far more specific – must be the actual causal mechanism of depression. I suggest that this 'something else' most likely has to do with the brain mechanisms that actually generate depressive *feelings*.

Depression itself

My reason for suggesting this is the fact that the clinical *phenomenology* of depression is characterized, above all else, by a complex of feelings: low mood, low self-esteem, loss of motivation and energy, guilt, loss of pleasure in the world, and so on. Is this complex of feelings not the most obvious place to seek the essential nature of depression? And dare we ask whether this constellation of feelings means anything? It is after all in the essential nature of feelings that they mean something. It would be entirely normal and reasonable for all of us (even us scientists) to ask – outside of our scientific work – what it might mean when somebody says that they feel down, bad, defeated, useless; that they have lost all hope for themselves, lost all interest in other people, and so on. We would ask: *why* do they feel this? Certainly it is possible that the feelings are meaningless epiphenomena of depression – even though feelings are not normally meaningless – but it is at least equally possible (and in my view, more so) that they are not meaningless.

I think the most helpful way of making sense of this complex of feelings is suggested by the DSM IV definition of major depression described as diagnostic criterion E:

> The symptoms are not better accounted for by *bereavement* (emphasis added).

This differential diagnostic criterion suggests that depression may be easily mistaken for bereavement, which in turn suggests that depression is characterized by a complex of feelings that closely resembles those associated with grief. It therefore seems reasonable to infer that depression might have something to do with social *loss*. This reminds us of what the early psychological investigators of depression (who were not embarrassed by feelings and their meanings) concluded on the basis of talking to patients about what their depression might mean to them personally: they concluded that depression was akin to *grief*, that it seemed in fact to be a pathological form of *mourning* (Freud, 1917).[2]

It is in fact well established today that early separation experiences do indeed predispose to depression (Heim & Nemeroff, 1999; Pryce et al., 2005), possibly through mediation of the stress cascades that McEwan (2000) has identified, and possibly also via other 'general sickness' mechanisms (McEwen, 2007). We also know that a first depressive episode is most likely to be triggered by social loss (Bowlby, 1980), and so on.

Affective neuroscience

In light of such commonplace observations to the effect that depressive feelings are connected with the psychology of attachment and loss, why are cognitive neuroscientists not focusing their attention on the mammalian brain systems that evolved specifically for the purpose of mediating attachment and loss, and which produce the particular type of pain associated with these biological phenomena of universal significance, namely separation distress (also known as 'protest' or 'panic') which, if it does not result in reunion, is typically followed by hopeless 'despair'?

It is well established that a specific mammalian brain system evolved precisely to generate these depression-like feelings (Panksepp, 1998, 2003, 2005). This brain system evolved from general pain mechanisms, millions of years ago, apparently for the purpose of forging long-term attachments between mothers and their offspring, between sexual mates, and ultimately between social groups in general. When such social bonds are broken through separation or loss of a loved one, or the like, then these brain mechanisms make the sufferer feel bad in a particular way. This special type of pain is called separation distress or panic. The biological value of this type of pain is that *it motivates the sufferer to avoid separation, and to seek reunion with the lost object*. However, if this biologically desirable outcome fails to materialize, then a second mechanism kicks in, which shuts down the distress and causes the lost individual to *give up*. This giving up is the 'despair' phase of social loss (Panksepp et al., 1989, 1991).

This system is embodied in a well-defined network of brain structures, starting in the anterior cingulate gyrus (about which so much has been said in recent neuro-imaging studies and deep brain stimulation treatments of depression; Mayberg et al., 2005), coursing downwards through various thalamic, hypothalamic and other basal forebrain nuclei, terminating in the ancient midbrain (pain generating) neurons of the periaqueductal grey. Activation and deactivation of this system is fundamentally mediated by opioid receptors. Mu opioid agonists, in particular, activate it in such a way as to generate feelings of secure well-being that are the very opposite of depression, whereas mu opioid blockade or withdrawal produces separation distress. This state is most readily identified in animal models by distress vocalizations (Panksepp, 1998). Bowlby (1980) classically described this phenotype as 'protest' behaviour, which he contrasted with the more chronic 'despair' behaviours that immediately follow on from it. The transition from acute 'protest' to chronic 'despair' presumably evolved to protect the separated animal from metabolic exhaustion, or alternatively to deflect the attention of predators, or both. In other words, *it positively motivates the animal to give up*.

It is the 'despair' phenotype that seems most closely to resemble clinical depression (Harris, 1989). The separation distress system, which is greatly sensitized by the floods of hormones (oestrogen, progesterone) and peptides (prolactin, oxytocin) that precede childbirth and facilitate maternal care, developed early in mammalian evolution. This is why the mechanisms which mediate attachment and separation are much more sensitive in *females* – who are more than twice as likely as males to suffer from depression. How do serotonin theorists account for this significant fact?

We have also known for a long time that the chemicals that mediate the brain's separation/attachment mechanism (opioids) have powerful anti-depressant properties (Bodkin et al., 1995). If it were not for the addictive risks of opiates, they would almost certainly have formed the front line of anti-depression medications. In fact, there is good reason to believe that the natural brain chemicals – endorphins – that make us feel good when we are safely and securely attached are themselves addictive; in short, that affectionate bonds are a primal form of addiction. This system apparently provides the elemental means by which mother and infant attach to each other – the means by which they become addicted to one another.

Although these opioid-driven attachment systems may be the pivotal mechanism in depression, there are many associated mechanisms that mediate the various depressive subtypes. For example, kappa opioid (dynorphin) facilitated shutdown of dopamine-driven appetitive systems (when an individual 'gives up' in despair) forms an independent aetiological mechanism in a majority of cases (Nestler & Carlezon, 2006).

It seems that the pain of social loss and defeat are the price that we mammals had to pay for the evolutionary advantages bestowed by this system, that is, by mammalian social attachment, the prototype of which is the mother–infant bond. This is an instance of a more general principle: conscious feelings, both positive and negative, evolved because they enhance survival and reproductive success. This is their causal role.

Neuropsychoanalysis

The evolutionary processes that gave rise to such emotional endophenotypes do not coincide with their higher cortical representations, let alone with their experiential end-products.

An infant in the grip of separation distress does not consciously think: "this loss of my beloved mother is bad for me because it endangers my survival and thereby reduces my reproductive fitness". What the individual feels may *ultimately* serve the interests of the species, but the individual organism experiences only itself, not the biological mechanisms that gave rise to it. The infant simply feels bad, and then thinks something like: "this loss of my beloved mother is bad; I want her back". Or it feels: "This loss of my mother is bad; I hate it ... so I hate her."

Individuals are motivated primarily by subjective feelings, and secondarily by subjective thoughts; not by objective mechanisms. This is true even if the objective mechanisms *explain* the subjective feelings and thoughts in question. Here is a more complex example: the objective mechanism of the 'despair' phase of the separation response appears to be a shutdown of the 'protest' phase, with its associated *seeking* impulses. This prevents metabolic exhaustion, the risk of attracting predatory interest and the dangers of straying too far. At the neurochemical level this shutdown is probably mediated by dynorphin blockade of dopamine arousal, which (in behaviourist terms) replaces positive approach behaviours with negative withdrawal behaviours. In learning-theory terms: the seeking of 'rewards' elicits 'punishment' responses. This also involves frustration of SEEKING desires, which normally elicits *rage* responses (Panksepp, 1998). The *rage* responses must therefore be inhibited, or even reversed. Subjectively, this mechanism is reflected in the fact that hope is replaced by hopelessness, leading to anhedonia, or worse: hope is replaced by an attack on the self. The subjective outcome is thus quite different from the objective mechanism: "shut down *seeking* to promote survival" becomes "I hate the part of me that needs her and hopes she will come back" (cf. the so-called 'negative therapeutic reaction').

The fact that such a process might, at the representational (neocortical) level, involve an attack upon an internalized frustrating object is neither here nor there. The objective mechanism which explains (and ultimately causes) this state of affairs is the survival advantage of a shift from 'protest' to 'despair'. The subjective experience of this shift – a loss of self-esteem or worse: self-hatred – is entirely ignorant of the underlying mechanism, *but it motivates the organism to behave in the way that it does.*

I'm not suggesting drugs or deep brain stimulation are the way we should treat depression, but the drugs that actually work *prove the concept.* This is why it is interesting to be able to report that, recently, Panksepp and colleagues (Coenen et al., 2011) have developed a successful surgical intervention for intractable major depression by inserting a deep brain stimulator directly into the *seeking* system, thereby reversing the separation distress shutdown response described above. Likewise, he and colleagues (Yovell et al., 2016) successfully treated suicidal patients with Buprenorphine, the relatively safe opiate that Bodkin used (see above), which acts directly on the *panic* system. And he had dramatic results. None of his patients killed themselves, their mood lifted, and this was sustained over the period of time that he studied them. It made sense to use Buprenorphine on these patients, not only because suicidality clearly has more to do with the 'protest' phase of the separation distress cascade, but also because ethically in such cases you can't sit around for three weeks waiting for SSRIs to work – if they do work.

We neuropsychoanalysts are therefore formulating hypotheses which have led to the development of neurosurgical and psychopharmacological treatments – arising out of an understanding that these feelings in the symptom complex called depression *mean* something; that depression arises in relation to a specific kind of social context, a biological situation of universal significance. The brain chemistries mediating these brain circuits therefore mean something too. They respond to a particular social situation, a particular psychological constellation, a particular type of object relation (loss). That is what triggers this mechanism. The power of the neuropsychoanalytical approach is that the gap between a psychopharmacological understanding and a psychotherapeutic understanding is reduced dramatically. They don't become competing ways of understanding what is going on; they just become alternative ways of treating what is going on – complementary ways of treating what is going on. We should also recall that not all patients are amenable to psychoanalysis, especially not chronically depressed and suicidal patients.

Conclusion

So why does depression feel bad? It feels bad, according to affective neuroscience and neuropsychoanalysis, for two reasons: firstly, to encourage us to form attachments, particularly to early care-giving figures, but also with our sexual mates and offspring and social groups and the like; and secondly, to persuade us to give up hope if our attempts to reunite with such figures or groups do not succeed within a limited time frame, when we have become detached (or lost). The aetiological fact that such feelings can be too easily provoked, or too difficult to erase, etc., in some individuals, is immaterial to the biological forces that selected them into the mammalian genome in the first place.

In light of the existence of brain structures that generate such feelings, it seems reasonable to at least hypothesize that the linchpin of depression is none of the things that have so preoccupied contemporary psychiatric researchers over the past three decades, but rather the evolutionarily conserved brain state that mediates the transition from 'protest' to 'despair' in the wake of social loss. In other words, it seems reasonable to hypothesize that the core brain basis of depression revolves around the process by which separation distress is normally shut down (possibly by kappa-opioids like dynorphin), prompting the animal to 'give up'.

Why aren't mainstream psychiatric researchers investigating the role of these candidate brain processes in depression? They seem to be the obvious place to start, if we are going to take the phenomenology of depression itself (as opposed to things that correlate with it) as our starting point – as we in neuropsychoanalysis have.

We believe that such obvious starting points are neglected due to an ongoing, deep prejudice against acknowledging the implications for science of the subjective nature of feelings, and their causal efficacy in the brain. This prejudice is most unfortunate, because subjective feelings certainly exist, and they almost certainly evolved for a reason (they almost certainly enhanced reproductive fitness).

Feelings are, accordingly, almost certainly a central feature of how the brain works. We therefore ignore them at our peril.

Notes

1 It is important to note, though, that even this step is disallowed by many scientists when it comes to non-human animals. It is still widely considered anthropomorphist to infer conscious states from the behaviour of animals who cannot verbally 'declare' their feelings. How can they seriously believe that feelings are uniquely human, that affect emerged in evolution only with the appearance of human beings!
2 Freud used the term '*Trauer*', which Strachey translated as 'mourning' but which can also be translated as 'grief'.

References

Berger, M., Gray, J. A., Roth, B. L. (2009). The expanded biology of serotonin. *Annual Review of Medicine*, 60, 355–366.

Bodkin, J. A., Zornberg, G. L., Lukas, S. E., & Cole, J. O. (1995). Buprenorphine treatment of refractory depression. *Journal of Clinical Psychopharmacology*, 15, 49–57.

Bowlby, J. (1980). *Loss: Sadness and depression*. New York, NY: Basic Books.

Coenen, V. A., Schlaepfer, T. E., Maedler, B., & Panksepp, J. (2011) Cross-species affective functions of the medial forebrain bundle-implications for the treatment of affective pain and depression in humans. *Neuroscience and Biobehavioural Reviews*, 35, 1971–1981.

De Kloet, E., Joels, M. , & Holsboer, F. (2005). Stress and the brain: From adaptation to disease. *Nature Reviews Neuroscience*, 6, 463–475.

Delgado, P. L., Charney, D. S., Price, L. H., Aghajanian, G. K., Landis, H., & Heninger, G. R. (1990). Serotonin function and the mechanism of antidepressant action: Reversal of antidepressant-induced remission by rapid depletion of plasma tryptophan. *Archives of General Psychiatry*, 47, 411–418.

Freud, S. (1917). Mourning and melancholia. *Standard Edition*, 14: 239–258. London: Hogarth Press.

Freud, S. (1940). An outline of psychoanalysis. *Standard Edition*, 23: 144–207. London: Hogarth Press.

Harris, J. C. (1989). Experimental animal modeling of depression and anxiety. *Psychiatric Clinics of North America*, 18, 815–836.

Harro, J., & Oreland, L. (2001). Depression as a spreading adjustment disorder of monoaminergic neurons: A case for primary implications of the locus coeruleus. *Brain Research Reviews*, 38, 79–128.

Heim, C., & Nemeroff, C. (1999). The impact of early adverse experiences on brain systems involved in the pathophysiology of anxiety and affective disorders. *Biological Psychiatry*, 46, 1509–1522.

Koziek, M., Middlemas, D., & Bylund, D. (2008). Brain-derived neurotrophic factor and its receptor tropomyosin-related kinase B in the mechanism of action of antidepressant therapies, *Pharmacology & Therapeutics*, 117, 30–51.

Levinson, D. F. (2006). The genetics of depression: A review. *Biological Psychiatry*, 60, 84–92.

Mayberg, H., Lozano, A., Voon, V., McNeely, H., Seminowicz, D., Hamani, C., Schwalb, J., & Kennedy, S. (2005). Deep brain stimulation for treatment-resistant depression. *Neuron*, 45, 651–660.

McEwen, B. S. (2000). The neurobiology of stress: From serendipity to clinical relevance. *Brain Research*, 886(1–2), 172–189.

McEwen, B. S. (2007). Physiology and neurobiology of stress and adaptation: Central role of the brain. *Physiological Reviews*, 87, 873–904.

Nestler, E. J., & Carlezon, W. A. Jr. (2006). The mesolimbic dopamine reward circuit in depression. *Biological Psychiatry*, 59, 1151–1159.

Panksepp, J. (1998). *Affective neuroscience: The foundations of human and animal emotion*. New York: Oxford University Press.

Panksepp, J. (2003). Feeling the pain of social loss. *Science*, 302, 237–239.

Panksepp, J. (2005). Feelings of social loss: The evolution of pain and the ache of a broken heart. In: R. Ellis & N. Newton (Eds), *Consciousness & emotions* (Vol. 1. pp. 23–55). Amsterdam: John Benjamins.

Panksepp, J., Lensing, P., & Bernatzky, G. (1989). Delta and kappa opiate receptor control of separation distress. *Neuroscience Abstracts*, 15, 845.

Panksepp, J., Yates, G., Ikemoto, & Nelson, E. (1991). Simple ethological models of depression: Social-isolation induced "despair" in chicks and mice. In: B. Olivier & J. Moss (Eds.), *Animal Models in Psychopharmacology* (pp. 161–181). Holland: Duphar.

Pryce, C. R., Ruedi-Bettschen, D., Dettling, A. C., Weston, A., Russig, H. Ferger, B., & Feldon, J. (2005). Long-term effects of early-life environmental manipulations in rodents and primates: Potential animal models in depression research. *Neuroscience and Biobehavioral Reviews*, 29, 649–674.

Sacks, O. (1984). *A leg to stand on*. New York, NY: Picador.

Schildkraut, J. (1965) The catecholamine hypothesis of affective disorders: a review of supportive evidence. *American Journal of Psychiatry*, 122, 509–522.

Solms, M. (2018). The scientific standing of psychoanalysis. *British Journal of Psychiatry International*, 15, 5–8.

Solms, M., & Panksepp, J. (2010). Why depression feels bad. In: E. Perry, D. Collerton, F. LeBeau & H. Ashton (Eds.), *New horizons in the neuroscience of consciousness*. Amsterdam: John Benjamins.

Watt, D. & Panksepp, J. (2009). Depression: An Evolutionarily Conserved Mechanism to Terminate Separation Distress? A Review of Aminergic, Peptidergic, and Neural Network Perspectives. *Neuropsychoanalysis*, 11, 7–51.

Yovell, Y., Bar, G., Mashiah, M., Baruch, Y., Briskman, I., Asherov, J., Lotan, A., Rigbi, A., & Panksepp, J. (2016). Ultra-low-dose Buprenorphine as a time-limited treatment for severe suicidal ideation: A randomized controlled trial. *The American Journal of Psychiatry*, 173, 491–498.

Zellner, M., Watt, D., Solms, M., & Panksepp, J. (2011). Affective neuroscientific and neuropsychoanalytic approaches to two intractable psychiatric problems: Why depression feels so bad and what addicts really want . *Neuroscience & Biobehavioral Reviews*, 35, 2000–2008.

Zupancic, M., & Guilleminault, C. (2006). Agomelatine: A preliminary review of a new antidepressant. *CNS Drugs*, 20, 981–992.

16 Thoughts on the failure of intersubjective development following maternal–child trauma and loss

Daniel S. Schechter

The case of Lea

In her conclusion to the case of her patient, Lea, Dr. Kratel alludes to a paper and book by César and Sara Botella (2007), *La Figurabilité Psychique* (Psychic figurability (i.e. representation), in noting that the patient "carries away with his/her gaze turned inward, mother's gaze. This is the development of auto-eroticism—i.e. the pleasure in fantasy of receiving the admiring regard of the other". In so doing, what matters is "the ability of the child to reproduce … at the sensorimoter level, what he/she feels when being seen by mother". Dr. Kratel points out the possible relationship of this psychological phenomenon with Vittorio Gallese's discussion of the mirror neurons and the "birth of intersubjectivity" very early in development as described in his New York lectures "From Mirror Neurons to Embodied Simulation: A New Perspective on Intersubjectivity" from 2010 (available on YouTube).

We then note—as in the case of Kratel's Lea—that a failure of this launching of intersubjectivity between the child and the (m)other likely make it difficult to separate and individuate. And so one is left in the schizoid–paranoid position in Kleinian terms. As she says, "the object's great need becomes unbearable, the object hates this need, and this hatred must be extruded or projected such that 'I need his/her love' becomes 'he/she hates me, he/she is persecuting me'".

This view indeed resonates with a particular clinical dilemma for child analysts and psychotherapists when we find one or both parents are traumatized, suffering from depression and/or post-traumatic stress. The development of secondary intersubjectivity is blocked. I have written about this particular constellation and would like to thus present to you an excerpt of my paper "And then there was intersubjectivity: Addressing child self and mutual dysregulation during traumatic play" which was published in the Louis Sander Memorial Issue of *Psychoanalytic Inquiry* in 2019. This paper integrates what I have learned from our own empirical research on the effects of maternal post-traumatic stress related to interpersonal violence on the infant–mother relationship but also provides some very practical clinical techniques that I have developed from my own clinical and clinical research observations.

DOI: 10.4324/9781003279297-16

Excerpt from "And then there was intersubjectivity"

In his landmark paper, "Paradox and Resolution" (1997), Lou Sander presented what he termed as two "biological givens" (p. 153): (1) self-regulation and (2) the capacity for parent–infant synchrony and attunement. The latter is akin to the concept of "mutual regulation" that was coined by Gianino and Tronick (1986, p. 5) in their efforts to extend Sander's original ideas (Condon & Sander, 1974), a concept that has played a central role in my own research (Schechter et al., 2010). Sander argued that these two biological givens, furthermore, form the foundation for an individual's capacity to self-organize, to experience a sense of agency, to tolerate aloneness, and to love and be loved. And he further pointed out that psychopathology in the course of early childhood development could originate with difficulties in either or both of these biological givens. Both the innate drive toward self-regulation and that toward mutual regulation between self and other are continuously operating, parallel and simultaneous processes that can lend to tension, which can be experienced both as stressful and as pleasurable. The individual is forever seeking to strike a balance between self- and mutual-regulation, and, as Sander himself said, "through mutual modification, [the self–other system can transiently] reach harmonious coordination" (Sander, 1977, p. 138). He spoke of the analogy to the physics of two vibrating bodies such as tuning forks, each with their individual pitch, which when placed in proximity, can interface and resonate with one another or clash (Sander, 2002).

Sander asserted that, as self- and mutual regulation are non-cognitive processes, the fluctuation of the degree of resonance, of harmony between self- and mutual regulation and their interaction, leaves traces in the procedural (implicit), rather than declarative memory. Past moments, outside of conscious awareness, inform but cannot reliably determine the present interaction. This margin of uncertainty is consistent with non-linear dynamic systems theory to which Sander ascribed.

Karlen Lyons-Ruth and the Boston Change Process Group (Lyons-Ruth et al., 1998) later defined the term implicit relational knowing as a form of such procedural memory traces regarding being able to anticipate interaction patterns with intimate others based on prior experience with that individual—or as Daniel Stern has called this, "the schema of being with another in a certain way" (Stern, 1995, p. 93). As Lyons-Ruth et al. (1998) wrote, "A moment of meeting is the transactional event that rearranges the patient's implicit relational knowing by rearranging the intersubjective field between patient and therapist" (pp. 285–286). Sander described the specific recognition of the other's subjective reality as a prerequisite for such a moment of meeting to take place.

I assert that if the child's subjective state and striving toward intersubjective states with the traumatized mother must be avoided by her to maintain her psychobiological homeostasis in the wake of trauma, the moment of meeting cannot take place. Indeed, in our empirical research, we have shown that the helpless state of mind of the infant and young child, such as during a laboratory separation of mother from child, is enough to trigger significant psychobiological dysregulation of mothers who have been exposed to interpersonal violence during childhood and later in life and who have developed post-traumatic stress disorder (PTSD) related to their violent experiences. Compared to mothers without PTSD, these traumatized mothers show significantly less medial prefrontal cortical activity and greater limbic activity in response to watching videotapes of their toddlers during separation as compared to during free-play (Schechter et al., 2012). It is as if these mothers are decorticated and turn to a mode of survival that favors auto-regulation over mutual regulation and social affiliation (Porges, 2007). Mothers with PTSD related to violence also show characteristically different patterns of autonomic nervous system response to mother–child separation stress (Schechter et al., 2014).

These biological data converge with our behavioral findings, as we have shown that it is precisely in the wake of the mother–child separation task in the lab that mothers who develop PTSD following direct experiences of physical or sexual abuse or assault from childhood onward or who were exposed as witnesses to domestic violence during childhood—and thus who have what we call interpersonal violence-related post-traumatic stress disorder (IPV-PTSD)—as compared to non-PTSD controls, are less available to their toddlers for joint attention when the child makes a social bid to the mother (Schechter et al., 2010). Mothers who develop IPV-PTSD have symptoms of re-experiencing, avoidance/numbing, and hyperarousal that develop in the wake of exposure to physical and/or sexual abuse or assault from childhood through adulthood. We have also shown that IPV-PTSD mothers particularly tend to be more withdrawn and avoidant during reunion with their children, as well as more generally in their caregiving behavior (Schechter et al., 2008). And thus, the specific recognition of her child's subjective reality fails to take place. This leads to greater self-dysregulation in the child, as we showed in a follow-up study of the children of mothers with PTSD using the MacArthur Story-Stem Battery (Schechter et al., 2007).

The child's job

The infant and young child—in the face of an unpredictable, dysregulated, and dysregulating caregiving environment presented by a violence-exposed mother with PTSD—has the job before him of adapting to this environment to maintain a relationship with her, so as to ensure survival and to feel her emotional presence. The child thus must enter into the traumatized parent's intersubjective world and attempt to harmonize with her hyper-aroused state or, in a reversal of roles, attempt to modulate it in order to hold his parent's attention (Schechter et al., 2017). Even if the child experiences no violent events, he can be exposed vicariously to aspects of his mother's trauma through her behavior in response to traumatic memory traces to which he has no access. Her nonverbal behavior will—as in a game of Charades—communicate one or more aspects of her traumatic experience. In response, the child will interpret his mother's communication, yet without his mother's frame of reference or her adult capacity to make coherent narrative sense of her behavior. In turn, the child's uninformed, developmentally limited interpretation and resultant behavioral response may well have an effect on his mother and her emotional regulation, leading to a perpetually changing variation on the original maternal memory trace that is only fully knowable to her. The resulting cost to the child's sense of self, to his social–emotional development, can be considerable if, through other relationships, his primary attachment figure permitting, he does not find alternative ways of being-with the other in the interest of the development of intersubjectivity, potential flexibility, and complexity in future relationships.

So, what happens when, as we see all too often in our clinical work, a child—on top of having a parent, a mother who has had an exposure to violence and has subsequently developed PTSD—is exposed to interpersonal violence and develops his or her own PTSD? Even if the child's parent has not herself been traumatized, addressing the needs of one's own child who has experienced violent trauma, coping with the disruption to a sense of safety and a need for its restoration, the accompanying emotional pain, possible sense of shame, and terrifying memory traces—not to forget the disturbance to self-regulation and physiologic homeostasis—can all be very challenging. Typically, the parent and child must cope with the child's feeling that there was a failure of protection with accompanying guilt, sadness, and anger on the part of the non-offending parent. Now if the parent also has a history of being a victim and/or witness of violent trauma and suffers from related PTSD too, there might, on the one hand, be an opportunity for greater empathy, reflection, and efforts at making meaning of the trauma, given her possible understanding of what it is like to have lived through a similarly threatening event. The latter is particularly true if the parent has had the benefit of a positive, secure attachment and, thus, a model for self- and mutual regulation. Yet, all too often we find that this is not the case, at least not without focused intervention (Schechter et al., 2015).

The parent's PTSD and accompanying emotional dysregulation, which are all too often part of an intergenerational process, are rather triggered by helpless states of mind, aggressive gestures as reminders of traumatic events even in the child's play. The post-traumatic re-experiencing, avoidance, hyperarousal, and/or dissociation, the accompanying emotional dysregulation can well foreclose the possibility of parental openness to receive the child's emotional communication, bids for joint attention, and striving for intersubjective joining and meaning-making (Schechter et al., 2010). In turn, the child's post-traumatic re-experiencing often manifested as traumatic re-enactment in play, his anxious avoidance, and hyperarousal and/or dissociation and numbing, as well as his possibly increased aggression toward self via self-endangering behavior or other, are all possible adaptations of the dysregulated (i.e., traumatized) child to being with the dysregulated (i.e., traumatized) and dysregulating (traumatizing) parent. It is most often the traumatized parent who identifies a problem, which is most often perceived as residing in the child and causing distress and/or dysfunction in the parent (Schechter et al., 2012).

These critical moments, I assert, must be seized by the therapist in the caregiver's presence to help the dyad out of a mutually helpless and/or hostile, mutually dysregulated state. For the child, the therapist catalyzes a moment of connection with the parent that has been heretofore avoided, and thus validates the child's experience and forges a path to his experience of being known by the therapist and caregiver in an effort of joint attention to the child's emotional communication. For the parent, the therapist's curiosity about and openness to receiving the child's communication provides support and a model for this impaired function on the part of the parent and a source of mutual regulation between the therapist and the parent at a moment of heightened stress in the parent–child dyad. This support, modeling, and opportunity for mutual therapist–parent regulation can contribute to a greater sense of parental competence in the face of a crippling parental sensation of helplessness.

Such moments of meeting are often most ripe during traumatic play, during which the child is seemingly compelled to re-experience and re-enact one or more sequences of the experience that overwhelmed him (Gaensbauer, 1995; Coates, 2016).

A new clinical vignette

At this point, I would like to offer a never before published case example that extends what I have described above in the excerpt from "And then there was intersubjectivity" (Schechter, 2019), to illustrate and extend its thesis. It is the case of a little girl, Dalila, and her mother, Anne-Marie, who agreed to my sharing the following anonymized vignette.

Dalila was a blonde nearly 4-year-old girl who entered my office with wide eyes as if at once frightened and excited to find herself with her mother and me in my consulting room with so many colorful toys on display. Her mother had called to ask for a consultation as she was concerned about the effects on Dalila of domestic violence by Dalila's father and the abrupt move to a domestic violence shelter and measures of no-contact with police report that had been put in place. Dalila's mother Anne-Marie was a native French-speaking Swiss woman originally of Protestant faith who had married an Algerian Islamic man and converted to his faith. While he obliged her to remain a strict follower of Islam, he binge drank hard liquor and abused cocaine and cannabis, in the context of likely untreated bipolar disorder and a history of physical abuse as a child in Algeria. Anne-Marie appeared for the first visit in my office in full burka with face covering and avoided eye contact with me. Anne-Marie described florid post-traumatic stress disorder symptoms related to being hit, pushed, nearly strangled, with regular threats to her life. She had flashbacks and intrusive memories, severe insomnia, with nightmares when she did sleep. She experienced panic when she saw any man who resembled her husband, and when the public bus passed by his or his sister's apartment, for fear that he might see her or find out where she lived or was going. She experienced hypervigilance to sounds and double-checked the locks, hallways, and sidewalks when entering and leaving her shelter. Anne-Marie disclosed that her husband had also lost his temper with Dalila, had screamed that she was a "little slut like her mother" and had slapped her across the face, hit her arm, and briskly shaken her when she had a temper tantrum or spoke too loudly. He had also pushed Dalila out of the way as the little girl had tried to protect her mother. Despite these allegations, Dalila had not been left with physical traces of injury. Yet she was clearly scared of her father while also missing him as he had the tendency unexpectedly to surprise her with gifts and cuddles or give her cookies when she did not expect it.

During the first consultation I noted Dalila did not explore the many toys that were visible on the shelves and around the perimeter of the carpeted play area. She remained very vigilant, darting glances towards her mother and then towards me. Yet she was careful to keep her distance from me as if showing me the confusion and wariness she experienced with her father, and stayed rather close to her mother, almost as if hiding behind her. She would go on in later sessions to turn this into a game, hiding under her mother's burka or under a blanket and pillows I had in a corner, and waiting to surprise me.

Meanwhile, Dalila expressed herself well and interacted in play throwing a ball in my direction that I returned, and then rolling cars my way, even though contact was fleeting and distance maintained. Her mother said that Dalila had not wanted to come to a doctor because doctors are scary. I explained that I am not a doctor who gives shots. At that point, her mother helped Dalila turn towards me as she had buried her head in her mother's lap as she sat down. Her mother encouraged Dalila to show me some toys she had in her little backpack. Dolls and Playmobil figures. Dalila then told a little story involving two girl characters, the big one was her "auntie" and the little one was a girl her same age. I asked where the mother and father were. Dalila answered with a scream and a look of rage, "No!" which she said several times before answering questions again from her mother. Her mother looked at me with tears in her eyes and said, "that's her father's voice—I can't stand it when she yells at me in that voice. It's like he's here—and I cry and I freeze. She suddenly has so much power. I become frightened!"

Anne-Marie was finally even more concerned, given Dalila's many contradictory behaviors. Anne-Marie revealed at that point her own history of trauma with a bipolar mother who during her early childhood had not yet been stabilized on medication and had behaved erratically and at times violently or seductively. Anne-Marie froze when her daughter would enact certain behaviors that Anne-Marie identified with her husband's violence. She described feeling paralyzed, helpless, and fearful at once of her daughter's harming her and of her losing control and possibly harming her daughter—

even though she stated that she had never lifted a finger to hit or threaten to hit Dalila.

Dalila then played out the scenario of going to the doctor and took the toy medical kit down from the shelf. She said that the little girl doll had a stomach ache from eating too much cake and said her arm hurt because someone hit it. This allowed me to open the field of why Dalila came to me with her mother. Using a family of lion figurines to play out a scene of conflict, I said interrogatively that I had heard that sometimes the daddy lion got very angry and said mean things and even hit the mommy, did that ever happen in your family? Dalila said "yes." I asked if she could remember one of those times and tell me about it. She became anxious and ignored the question, turning to continue her play. Her mother gave her an example of a time when Dalila annoyed her father by jumping on his lap to give him a kiss when he came home. Then she asked, "Did he hit you after that?" Dalila nodded affirmatively with gaze averted, and then she quickly changed the subject by asking her mother for a bun to eat which she ate ferociously as if she were turning into a lion. I said that it seemed to me that Dalila wanted to change the subject because she doesn't want to think about Daddy when he is threatening and that she was becoming a hungry lion. With that Dalila took the male lion figure and went up to her mother and roared and pretended to strike out at her mother with her hand-turned-paw. Her mother looked at me, saying, "See, what do I do now?" rather helplessly. I said, "As long as we are all playing, it is safe, let's see how the story evolves—maybe it's important for Dalila to know that we can find a way to stop the hungry lion from hurting everyone since that is so very scary." At that point, the mother feigned fear and said, "I'm going to call the zoo police and say that one hungry lion needs to go back in his cage before he hurts someone." I smiled and nodded to encourage this empowerment of the mother. Dalila said, "No one can stop me." I played the role of the zoo police and I said, "Lion, here is a big steak; and if you want to eat it, you have to come in this other cage. It's very delicious and juicy, the steak." With that, Dalila let her lion be locked in the other cage and she then switched to the role of the lion cub who hides under the chair and asks, "Is he gone?" The mother then went to find Dalila and cuddled with her, saying, yes, we're safe now! In this way, mother and child were able to co-construct a moment of repair in which a traumatic memory trace with the violent father was rendered accessible through play, in the presence of the regulating and mentalizing therapist, such that the mother was able to share intersubjectively in what Sander would have described as a moment of meeting, having contained the scary hungry lion in the room.

Conclusion

This chapter, based on my paper from 2019, has taken as its departure point the interference posed by violent trauma and associated parent–child psychopathology to self- and mutual regulation of emotion and arousal. Lou Sander drew a parallel between the capacity to engage in mutual regulation and the formation of intersubjective states during which moments of meeting arise. Our clinical experience and research have shown how violent traumatization can make the parent unable to receive the child's efforts towards intersubjectivity. PTSD can render the traumatized parent blind, deaf, senseless to her child's emotional communication, particularly when it triggers helpless states of mind that stir up traumatic memories. The child cannot depend on such a parent to help make sense of the present moment, as the parent remains hostage to her traumatic past.

The clinical examples in this article (of which I have presented one of two here) illustrate how the child, in such a context, who has himself additionally been exposed to violence, will, in the absence of a mutually regulating, inter-subjectively receptive caregiver, attempt to self-regulate through repetitive traumatic play.

This traumatic play can further alarm and distance the post-traumatically stressed caregiver such that the child and parent each become more dysregu-lated and then enter into a vicious circle of mutual dysregulation.

In addition to traumatic play, we have shown how the transmission of traumatic memory traces occur in daily, routine, parent–child interactions (i.e., separations and reunions) via "traumatically skewed intersubjectivity" (Schechter et al., 2017). As Sander stated long before,

> The simple repetitive situations that are a part of the daily life of mother and child in this early time of life should lend themselves admirably to a solid set of reliable anticipations about many dimensions of the mother's behavior.
>
> (Sander, 1977, p. 144)

Traumatic play is one form of such simple, repetitive behavioral manifestation of trauma-related memory traces within an intersubjective space shared by both caregiver and therapist. The addition of the therapist as an observing, reflecting third renders the traumatic memory traces open to updating and reconsolidation within that space (Stein, Rohde, & Henke, 2015). Updating and reconsolidation of the traumatic memory traces that incorporate the therapist's mentalizing stance, reassociation to previously avoided emotions (i.e., fear and helplessness), and the mutual regulatory process between therapist and traumatized parent and, in turn, parent and traumatized child, in a triadic constellation helps to extinguish fear and helplessness and offer shared meaning to what had been disconnected and nonsensical.

References

Botella, C., & Botella, S. (2007). *La figurabilité psychique.* Paris: Éditions in Press.

Coates, S. W. (2016). Can babies remember trauma? Symbolic forms of representation in traumatized infants. *Journal of American Psychoanalytic Association*, 64(4), 751–776.

Condon, W. S., & Sander, L. W. (1974). Synchrony demonstrated between movements of the neonate and adult speech. *Child Development*, 45(2), 456–464.

Gaensbauer, T. J. (1995). Trauma in the preverbal period: Symptoms, memories, and developmental impact. *Psychoanalytic Study of the Child*, 50, 122–149.

Gianino, A., & Tronick, E. Z. (1988). The mutual regulation model: The infant's self and interactive regulation coping and defense. In: T. Field, P. McCabe, & N. Schneiderman (Eds.), *Stress and coping* (pp. 47–68). Hillsdale, NJ: Erlbaum.

Lyons-Ruth, K., Bruschweiler-Stern, N., Harrison, A. M., Morgan, A. C., Nahum, J. P., Sander, L., Stern, D. N., & Tronick, E. Z. (1998). Implicit relational knowing: Its role in development and psychoanalytic treatment. *Infant Mental Health Journal*, 19(3), 282–289.

Porges, S. W. (2007). The polyvagal perspective. *Biological Psychology*, 74(2), 116–143.

Sander, L. (1997). Paradox and resolution: From the beginning. In: J. D. Noshpitz (Ed.), *Handbook of child and adolescent psychiatry*. New York, NY: Wiley.

Sander, L. (1977). The regulation of exchange in the infant-caretaker system and some aspects of the context-content relationship. In: M. Lewis & L. Rosenblum (Eds.), *Interaction, conversation, and the development of language* (pp. 133–156). New York, NY: Wiley.

Sander, L. (2002). Thinking differently: Principles of process in living systems and the specificity of being known. Psychoanalytic Dialogues, 12(1), 11–42.

Schechter, D. S. (2019). And then there was intersubjectivity: Addressing child self and mutual dysregulation during traumatic play. *Psychoanalytic Inquiry*, 39(1), 52–65.

Schechter, D. S., Coates, S. W., Kaminer, T., Coots, T., Zeanah, C. H., Davies, M., Schonfield, I. S., Marshall, R. D., Liebowitz, M. R., Trabka, K. A., McCaw, J., & Myers, M. M. (2008). Distorted maternal mental representations and atypical behavior in a clinical sample of violence-exposed mothers and their toddlers. *Journal of Trauma and Dissociation*, 9(2), 123–149.

Schechter, D. S., Moser, D. A., Aue, T., Gex-Fabry, M., Pointet, V. C., Cordero, M. I., Suardi, F., Manini, A., Vital, M., Sancho Rossignol, A., Rothenberg, M., Dayer, A. G., Ansermet, F., & Rusconi Serpa, S. (2017). Maternal PTSD and corresponding neural activity mediate effects of child exposure to violence on child PTSD symptoms. *PloS One*, 12(8), e0181066.

Schechter, D. S., Moser, D. A., McCaw, J. E., & Myers, M. M. (2014). Autonomic functioning in mothers with interpersonal violence-related posttraumatic stress disorder in response to separation-reunion. *Developmental Psychobiology*, 56(4), 748–760.

Schechter, D. S., Moser, D. A., Reliford, A., McCaw, J. E., Coates, S. W., Turner, J. B., Rusconi, S., & Willheim, E. (2015; epub February 20, 2014). Negative and distorted attributions towards child, self, and primary attachment figure, among posttraumatically stressed mothers: What changes with Clinical Assisted Videofeedback Exposure Sessions (CAVES)? *Child Psychiatry and Human Development*, 46(1), 10–20.

Schechter, D. S., Moser, D. A., Wang, Z., Marsh, R., Hao, X., Duan, Y., Yu, S., Gunter, B., Murphy, D., McCaw, J., Kangarlu, A., Willheim, E., Myers, M. M., Hofer, M. A., & Peterson, B. S. (2012). An fMRI study of the brain responses of traumatized mothers to viewing their toddlers during separation and play. *Social Cognitive and Affective Neuroscience*, 7(8), 969–979.

Schechter, D. S., Willheim, E., Hinojosa, C., Scholfield-Kleinman, K., Turner, J. B., McCaw, J., Zeanah, C. H., & Myers, M. M. (2010). Subjective and objective measures of parent–child relationship dysfunction, child separation distress, and joint attention. *Psychiatry: Interpersonal and Biological Processes*, 73(2), 130–144.

Schechter, D. S., Zygmunt, A., Coates, S. W., Davies, M., Trabka, K. A., McCaw, J., Kolodji, A., & Robinson, J. L. (2007). Caregiver traumatization adversely impacts young children's mental representations of self and others. *Attachment & Human Development*, 9(3), 187–205.

Stein, M., Rohde, K. B., & Henke, K. (2015). Focus on emotion as a catalyst of memory updating during reconsolidation. *Behavioral Brain Science*, 38, e27.

Stern, D. N. (1985). *The interpersonal world of the infant*. New York, NY: Basic Books.

Stern, D. N. (1995). *The motherhood constellation: A unified view of parent-infant psychotherapy*. New York, NY: Basic Books.

17 Containing darkness

Siri Erika Gullestad

Depression: the psychology of loss[1]

What does separation and loss do to us human beings? That was Bowlby's main question (Bowlby, 1969). When the child's desperate cry of protest – "Don't leave me! – is not heard, the result is despair. Prolonged despair may result in *detachment* – the child gets apathetic, stops seeking comfort – we remember the heart-breaking image of Little John in the film *Young Children in Brief Separations* by Joyce and James Robertson, lying quietly on the floor, sucking his thumb, embracing an enormous teddy bear. Detachment was identified through Bowlby's psychoanalytically informed perception: previously, the quiet child had been seen as a child that had adjusted to the unfamiliar environment of the hospital: "Little Maria does not cry any more, now she has adapted to the hospital setting" – that was how doctors and nurses understood the situation. Moreover, the message to the parents was: "We don't want you to visit. That will only disturb the child". So many children of my generation were left in hospitals without visits from their parents. I have seen many of them as patients. They come with permanent feelings of isolation, unrepresented despair, experiences of unreality. And they come with relational problems, unable to commit to intimate relationships: burnt child dreads the fire – they were once abandoned, helpless, and have promised themselves "never again". Rather the lonely road of self-sufficiency than being hurt once more.

There are three reasons why I emphasise this familiar story. The first is that Mark Solms' reference to the separation distress system that Bowlby identified and named gives me an opportunity to underline what a truly innovative scientific discovery the concept of detachment contains. As a psychoanalyst Bowlby saw "through" the adapted child; he saw a withdrawn child that had given up seeking contact. The recognition of detachment as an unconscious defence mechanism is a specifically psychoanalytic contribution to the understanding of the origin of psychopathology. The concept of detachment also highlights how systematic empirical observation goes hand in hand with theory development, i.e. conceptual research.

This reminder of the particular scientific contribution of psychoanalysis is of importance in times when many academic people doubt whether psychoanalysis

DOI: 10.4324/9781003279297-17

can be called a science. Psychoanalysis is not only a theory of treatment. It refers to a theory of personality – in psychology textbooks psychoanalysis is described as the most significant personality theory of the 19th century – and to a theory about psychopathology. Summing up, the psychoanalytic theory on attachment, separation, and loss is a contribution to the general science of psychology.

The second reason for emphasising detachment is that this advance in theoretical conceptualisation led to a revolution in practice, i.e. in the way small children are treated in hospitals. In Norway, the public health authorities, at the beginning of the 1970s, asked four psychologists and psychiatrists, among them two psychoanalysts, to write a report about children in hospital. This resulted in a small book called *Children Go to Hospital* (*Når barn må på sykehus*) (Auestad et al., 1973). On the basis of Bowlby's theory of attachment, separation, and loss, the book argues for a new practice, *rooming-in*, that allows parents to accompany their children and be with them in the hospital. Think how many depressions were prevented by this change in practice in the hospitalisation of children! In a time where prevention is what the public health system aims at, we should be proud of the extremely important contribution to prevention made by psychoanalytic attachment theory.

The third reason why I wanted to remind us of this story is Bowlby's fate in the psychoanalytic community – how his theory was received. Bowlby had hoped to contribute to the scientific development of psychoanalysis; what he experienced, however, was that much of the analytic world "closed ranks against him", as Grotstein has called it (Holmes, 1995). It was a time when many psychoanalysts did not appreciate real events – actual trauma – as a cause of psychopathology, and would not recognise the value of the empirical research that Bowlby brought to psychoanalysis. I thought that this resistance to empirical research was a bygone. When I see the critique, sometimes quite harsh, that neuropsychoanalysis is subject to, I feel a rush of ice-cold air from the past. Bowlby recognised the existence of the separation–distress system. Mark Solms demonstrates that this system has clear biological markers. A beautiful example of how psychoanalytic theory can be substantiated by neuroscience. That this research is not welcomed is depressing. If this attitude towards research gains dominance, the future of psychoanalysis is, as I see it, in danger.

The specific contribution of psychoanalysis

In 2003, the theme of the Sandler conference was depression. One of the main speakers was Hugo Bleichmar, who presented a paper called "Some subtypes of depression, their interrelations and implication for psychoanalytic treatment", based on his article in IJP from 1996. I was invited as a discussant of his paper – a discussion that was elaborated and published as an article in the *Scandinavian Psychoanalytic Review* (Gullestad, 2003). The point of departure for the article is that depression can be studied from many perspectives. In my 40-year long professional life as a professor of clinical psychology at the University of Oslo, I have been in dialogue with colleagues from different research and therapeutic traditions. At the psychology department at the University of Oslo, the research on depression in terms of *cognitive deficits* is especially strong. The bright students ask whether the psychoanalytic understanding of depression is different from the cognitive understanding. Does psychoanalysis have a specific contribution to the understanding of depression?

Phenomenology of depression

In his discussion of the melancholic state Freud focuses on the ego: the melancholic displays an "extraordinary diminution in his self-regard, an impoverishment of his ego on a grand scale" (Freud, 1917, p. 246). The depressed person sees herself as incapable of fulfilling her wishes and needs, and of attaining her goals. The state of *helplessness* and *hopelessness* is underlined as a key feature. Helplessness also comes forward as core concept in the account of depression in general academic psychology, underpinned by experiments. The depressed person does not believe she can influence people and situations (*learned helplessness*, Rosenhan & Seligman, 1984). The experience of "I" as an agent, of believing that you can make a difference, is at the heart of being human. Depression is not only a disorder of mood. It is a disorder of *mental agency* (Fonagy, et al., 2002).

According to the theory of learned helplessness a crucial determinant is the causal attribution, or explanation, the individual makes. Depressive people attribute failure to themselves ("I'm stupid") instead of focusing external factors (e.g. "the task was difficult"; "I had a bad day"). *Attributional style* is a useful concept, expressing how we understand the relationship between the world and ourselves. Certainly, ways of thinking is what we address in everyday psychoanalytic work. The contradiction often set up between the affective and the cognitive domain is artificial – as psychoanalysts we of course deal with cognition. Summing up, the account of depression on a descriptive, phenomenological level is a shared one.

The question of why

However, attributional style does not represent a satisfying answer to the question of why – why the person has come to think and feel the way she does. Everyone can agree that depression is about loss and unfulfilled needs and wishes. However, a distinct contribution by psychoanalysis, as compared with the cognitive model, is to emphasise that needs and wishes may be unconscious. In Freud's words, the melancholic "knows whom he has lost, but not what he has lost in him" (Freud, 1917, p. 245).

The psychoanalytic understanding of depression is now a multidimensional one, characterised by interacting determinants, both internal and external. The Freudian prototype of "guilty depression" represents only one of many pathways leading to depressive states. Other paths include, e.g. trauma, abandonment, and identification with depressive parents, and depression due to narcissistic disorders

(Bleichmar, 1996). Furthermore, psychoanalysis underlines the significance of needs that are not represented in words (Gullestad, 2003). Loss may occur at a stage of development where a mental representation of a specific object has not yet been established ("la chose", Kristeva, 1987). We are here dealing with a specific modality of depression, "le deuil blanc" (Green, 1983) characterised by *le négatif* – i.e. absence, emptiness. Mourning is made difficult because affects are invested in "la chose" – the thing beyond words.

In an article called "Beyond semantics" Killingmo (1995) states: "As affects isolated on a pre-verbal level are deprived of expression on a semantic–symbolic level, they are not likely to be modified by content of interpretation alone" (Killingmo, 1995, p. 125). In this regard, Killingmo emphasises the significance of *intonation*, of the quality of the speech sound of the analyst, in becoming emotionally available for patients in this depressive–existential mode of being.

Within a diverse research field, where depression is studied from different angles – i.e. in terms of cognitive deficits or as learned behaviour – the contribution of psychoanalysis is that depression is most usefully studied at the level of *psychological causation* (Gullestad, 2003). The psychoanalytic understanding of depressive states in terms of unconscious interpretation and meaning of experience represents a distinctive contribution to depression research. As I see it, psychoanalysis has a double-edged epistemological position. On the one hand, psychoanalysis needs to be in dialogue with other scientific disciplines, like developmental psychology, memory research, and neuroscience. On the other hand, psychoanalysis represents a depth psychological research method that is able to capture data that are not accessible by other methods.

Depression: a normal aspect of life

In Norway, two leading psychologists within the cognitive field (Berge & Repål, 2002) published a book about depression titled: *Thieves of happiness ("Lykketyvene")*. The book is interesting, because I think it expresses a certain zeitgeist. The first sentence of the book reads like this: "Depression is like a thief that steals your joy". Several points of principle are implied here. First, we note that depression is seen as an entity that is external to the subject – something alien. This is in line with a medical model, seeing depression as an "illness" that the individual "gets", is "struck by" or "suffers from". In sharp contrast is the psychoanalytic viewpoint, which sees depression in terms of the subject's unconscious intentions, as a specific, but meaningful reaction to loss.

Certainly, the way we speak about a phenomenon forms how we understand it. In this regard the very use of "depression" as a noun deserves being reflected upon. Schafer (1976), in his seminal reflection of the language of psychoanalysis, insists on the reifying consequences of applying categories to describe psychological phenomena. Although we probably cannot do without nouns and categories in our theory, we must not overlook the alienating effects of using expressions like "having a depression". Talking like this places us in a medical universe. In contrast, the verbal form of "being depressed" stays in touch with the consciously and unconsciously feeling and acting individual, which is the distinct mark of psychoanalysis.

A second implication of characterising depression as a "thief of happiness" is that a base line of happiness and joy seems to be assumed as the normal state of affairs. Of course no one will deny that loss, sadness, and mourning are part of every human life, and actually, general psychological textbooks are on a line with Freud's fundamental distinction between mourning as a normal reaction to loss and depression as a mourning process gone awry. Indeed, depression is often an expression of what Mitscherlich & Mitscherlich (1967) have called *Die Unfähigkeit zu trauern* – an inability to mourn. Nevertheless, I think it is precisely the distinction that Freud made that risks getting lost in our present-day culture, with a dominating ideal of "happy life". Is the increase in depressive conditions in our society at least partly due to an increased inclination to see sadness, loss of initiative etc. not as normal mourning reactions but as a kind of abnormal phenomenon? The point is important. A patient came to see me after having been on antidepressants for half a year. The medication had resulted in a general feeling of apathy; he had lost his "ups and downs" but had no feeling of vitality and no sexual pleasure. Initially, he had sought his doctor because he felt utterly miserable and dejected after his wife announced that she wanted to divorce. After asking him a lot of questions about his symptoms (whether he had problems getting up in the morning etc.), his doctor had concluded that he suffered from depression, and had prescribed antidepressants. When I talked to him, I asked him how he experienced talking with his doctor about the crisis with his wife. He answered: "He did not ask me". This case clearly illustrates the normative implications of diagnosis: affective reactions to life events are not treated as such, but are seen as a set of symptoms indicating an "illness" that has to be treated with medication. Certainly, we are confronted with a medicalisation of human life problems. In contrast, psychoanalysis emphasises processes of loss and mourning as part of normal development. Concepts like "disillusionment" and "depressive position" bear witness to that. Indeed, psychoanalysis sees the ability to contain pain, sadness, and melancholic states as an expression of emotional maturity.

In this perspective, the containment of dysphoric affect has an adaptive significance. A young doctor, a gifted and charming man, came to me primarily because of anxiety. His self-representation was characterised by splitting, either "king of the world" or "no good". During the psychoanalytic treatment, the feeling of being inferior and unworthy became stronger and stronger, memories emerged, connected to his father always having preferred his elder brother – and he felt that therapy made him worse. Everything felt hopeless. I said to him: "Yes, a part of you feels that everything is hopeless. That is a painful feeling. May be that feeling has been with you since long ago, but it has been too hurtful for you to recognise. Now you dare to feel it – and that means that we can work on it together". This type of comment may help the patient to own his affective states: "*This* is how I have felt it". Thus, the feeling of hopelessness can be integrated in the individual's self-representation, as a part of the *me* experience. Such ego strengthening interventions are likely to assist the patient in coping with his/her depression.

Also, mourning processes may be a precondition for creativity, as biographic studies of creative individuals have shown. From this perspective, the aim of psychoanalytic treatment of depression comes forward as radically different from that of cognitive therapy. Whereas the latter aims at correcting ways of thinking, psychoanalytic treatment aims at greater tolerance and integration of affective self-states – and of the dark side of life.

Note

1 Originally presented as a discussion of Mark Solms' paper *Neuropsychoanalysis of depression: Why depression feels bad.*

References

Auestad, A.M., Killingmo, B., Nyhus, H., & Pande, H. (1973). *Når barn må på sykehus* (*When children go to hospital*). Oslo: Universitetsforlaget.

Berge, T., & Repål, A. (2002). *Lykketyvene.* (*Thieves of happiness*). Oslo: Aschehoug.

Bowlby, J. (1969). Attachment. In *Attachment and loss.* New York: Basic Books.

Bleichmar, H. B. (1996). Some subtypes of depression and their implications for psychoanalytic treatment. *International Journal of Psychoanalysis*, 77, 935–961.

Bleichmar, H. B. (2003). *Some subtypes of depression, their interrelations and implications for psychoanalytic treatment.* Conference paper, Joseph Sandler Research Conference, University of Frankfurt, 2003.

Fonagy, P., Gergely, G., Jurist, E. L., & Target, M. (2002). *Affect regulation, mentalization, and the development of the self.* New York: Other Press.

Freud, S. (1917). Mourning and melancholia. *SE* 14. London: Hogarth Press.

Green, A. (1983). *Narcissisme de vie. Narcissisme de mort.* Paris: Lés Editions de Minuit.

Gullestad, S. E. (2003). One depression or many? *Scandinavian Psychoanalytic Review*, 26, 123–130.

Holmes, J. (1995). "Something there is that doesn't love a wall". John Bowlby, attachment theory, and psychoanalysis. In: S. Goldberg et al. (Eds.), *Attachment theory: Social development and clinical perspectives* (pp. 19–43). London: The Analytic Press.

Killingmo, B. (1990). Beyond semantics: A clinical and theoretical study of isolation. *International Journal of Psychoanalysis*, 71: 113–126.

Kristeva, J. (1987). *Soleil noir. Dépression et mélancholie.* Paris: Éditions Gallimard.

Mitscherlich, A., & Mitscherlich, M. (1967). *Die Unfähigkeit zu trauern.* München: Piper Verlag.

Rosenhan, D. L., & Seligman, M. E. P. (1984). *Abnormal psychology.* New York: W.W. Norton.

Schafer, R. (1976). *A new language for psychoanalysis.* New Haven, CT and London: Yale University Press.

Index